CONTENTS

1. INTRODUCTION

Pharmacovigilance is defined as the science of detection, assessment, and prevention of adverse effects of medicines.

Pharmacovigilance starts from the clinical trial stage and continues throughout the life cycle of the drug. The process of collection of safety information about a drug begins in phase one of the clinical trial, and continues after approval.

Clinical trials are carried out in a limited set of patients selected as per pre-determined inclusion – exclusion criteria. When a drug is approved after submission of the new drug application (NDA) physicians begin to prescribe it to the general population and a variety of patients in large number begin to take the drug. In such a scenario there may be adverse events that may be undetected in the preapproval pharmacovigilance (clinical trial reports) but may show up in the post approval pharmacovigilance. In the post approval phase several post-authorisation safety studies (PASS) are conducted. Some of these post marketing studies may be mandatory and may be required to be carried out as per policies of the national drug regulatory authority. In addition to such studies, spontaneous reports of adverse events also contribute to the post approval pharmacovigilance.

Pharmacovigilance therefore aims to monitor, identify and evaluate undesirable effects of drugs, and initiate measures to minimize the risk profile of the drugs. The objective of pharmacovigilance is to promote the safe and rational use of medicines and lead to improved patient care.

Pharmacovigilance is the science and activities relating to the detection, assessment, understanding and prevention of adverse effects or any other drug-related problems (WHO, 2002).

Pharmacovigilance activities include:

- lCollecting adverse event data
- lEvaluating the data with regard to safety
- lTaking decisions to protect public health
- lAnalyzing the results of action taken
- lCommunicating with stakeholders
- lCreating effective public awareness of the drug safety profile
- lMonitoring data to detect 'signals' (any new or changing safety issue)

Pharmacovigilance aims to enhance the effective use of medicines and prevent or minimize adverse events.

Those directly involved in pharmacovigilance include:

- lPatients who are the users of medicines
- lDoctors, pharmacists, nurses, clinical counselors and all other health care professionals working with medicines
- lRegulatory authorities
- lPharmaceutical companies (Sponsor)
- lCompanies importing or distributing medicines (Licensee of sponsor)

In 1968 the World Health Organisation (WHO) launched the global pharmacovigilance programme.

The objectives of this program are:

- lPrevention of unintended harm from the use of medicines.

- lSupport the analysis of risk versus benefit which in turn contributes to safer use of medicines.

- lImprovement in overall public health by the providing reliable information resulting in rational use of medicines.

2. NEED FOR PHARMACOVIGILANCE

Different patients differ in the manner they react to medicines. Variables such as medical history (contraindication) and concomitant medications (drug-drug interaction) can affect drug action and therapy outcomes. Brands of medicines differ in the manner in which they are produced and the ingredients and excipients that are used. The information we receive on the adverse effects of drugs in other countries may not be relevant. Ethnicity, genetic profile and physical characteristics can affect treatment modality.

In order to prevent unnecessary medical risk to the patient due to the inappropriate or unsafe use of medicines, monitoring system for the safety of medicines is required.

Extrapolation of data, to the U.K. National Health Service (NHS) revealed that, bed occupancy of patients admitted with adverse drug reactions (age group- above 16 years) could be as much as 5600 beds of the total NHS bed base.

In a study of the medicines used during pregnancy in Brazil, as many as 40% were not from the "approved drugs in pregnancy" and 3% were outright contraindicated.

Studies have revealed that around 5% of hospital admissions are due to an adverse drug reaction. In addition, there are adverse drug reactions caused by improper use of drugs such as overdose, drug abuse, as well as therapeutic failures due to lack of efficacy.

The number of spontaneous reports in the World Health Organization database was about 4.6 million reports in 2009, and this number was increasing by nearly 250,000 reports every year.

There is risk to patients from: Internet prescription, internet marketing, counterfeit medicines, substandard medicines and unapproved medicines.

The use of too many medicines per patient, inadequate dosage, use of antimicrobials in non-bacterial infection, injection use when oral formulations would suffice, failure to prescribe in accordance with clinical guidelines, self-medication, using prescription-only medicines without prescription, and use of higher antibiotics for minor conditions contribute to serious drug related issues. You can encounter skipped dose, medication error, missed dose, wrong prescription, and lack of efficacy with regards to medications.

Here is an example of a scam perpetrated by scamsters.

FDA WARNING

FDA ISSUES WARNING ON SCAM
A POTENTIALLY HARMFUL PRODUCT—REUMOFAN PLUS—IS BEING RELABELED AND SOLD UNDER THE NAME "WOW." IT'S BEING MARKETED TO TREAT ARTHRITIS, MUSCLE PAIN, OSTEOPOROSIS, BONE CANCER, AND OTHER CONDITIONS.

SOURCE: FDA WEBSITE.

To counteract all these risks there is a need for pharmacovigilance.

3. DEFINITIONS

Adverse Event

An adverse event (AE) is defined as any unfavorable and unintended sign including an abnormal laboratory finding, symptom, or disease associated with the use of a medicinal product, whether or not considered related to the medicinal product. Any untoward medical occurrence in a patient which does not necessarily have to have a causal relationship with this treatment.

An event is an adverse event whether or not it is considered as related to the medicinal product.

Examples:

After taking the suspect drug for a certain period the patient experienced dizziness, headache and asthenia.

After taking the suspect drug the patient experienced Chron's flare.

A pre-existing condition which, worsened in severity after administration of the product would also be considered as an adverse event.

Adverse Drug Reaction

In the pre-approval phase -- when therapeutic doses may not be established an adverse drug reaction is defined as: all noxious and unintended responses to the medicinal product at any dose.

In the pre-approval phase – clinical trial 1 - 3 – the drug is still under investigation and the dose may not be decided yet. Hence the definition states: at any dose.

In an adverse drug reaction, causality is a factor. A causal relationship between a medicinal product and an adverse event is at least a reasonable possibility, i.e., the relationship cannot be ruled out.

Serious Adverse Event

A serious adverse event (SAE) is any untoward medical occurrence that at any dose:

- Results in death.
Example: Cancer and tumors whose outcome is fatal. Completed suicide.

- 1 Is life-threatening.
The term "life-threatening" refers to an event in which the patient was at risk of death at the time of the event. It does not refer to an event which might have caused death if it were more severe at some future point.

Example: Status epilepticus, status asthmaticus, Steven Johnson syndrome.

- Requires inpatient hospitalization or prolongation of existing hospitalization.
Example: Gastro-intestinal hemorrhage, stroke.

- Results in persistent or significant disability/incapacity Example: Blindness, paralysis leading to inability to walk, amputation of limbs.

- Is a congenital anomaly or birth defect.
Example: Hydrocephalus, Anencephaly, atrial septal defect, tetralogy of fallot.

Another category of events that may be termed an SAE and require expedited reporting are Important Medical Events (IME). IME are events that may not fit in any of the above criteria but may jeopardize the medical condition of the patient or may require treatment to prevent one of the other outcomes listed above.

Examples of important medical events are angioneurotic oedema, episode of generalized tonic clonic seizure, oral contraception failure, drug withdrawal syndrome, and drug dependency. Lack of efficacy with a medicinal product used in treating life-threatening disease can also be an IME.

In the above examples you can see that the event of angioneurotic oedema can be managed in an emergency setting not resulting in hospitalization of more than 24 hours. The patient can be sent back home after being treated. An episode of generalized tonic clonic seizure would subside within minutes. Such events which require no hospitalization or do not fit into the six seriousness criteria, but are in themselves significant medical events are termed IME and categorized as SAE.

Expectedness of an Adverse Drug Event

Expected

If the reported event is present in the RSI it is considered to be expected. Unexpected An adverse event, the nature or severity of which is not consistent with the applicable product information - Investigator's Brochure for an unapproved investigational medicinal product and company core data sheet (CCDS) and summary of product characteristics (SmPC) for an approved product.

Investigator's Brochure, CCDS and SmPC constitute reference safety information (RSI).

An event is considered unexpected if it is:

A. Not present
B. More specific
C. More severe

Infection (listed in RSI) and the reported event is septicaemia. Septicaemia is a more specific condition and could be unexpected.

If the reported event is post traumatic stress disorder and the term in the RSI is stress, then again the event can be unexpected as it describes a more specific type of stress.

Convulsion (listed in RSI) and the reported term is status epilepticus. Here the term convulsions and status epilepticus differ in terms of severity and hence status epilepticus would be unexpected.

In applied pharmacovigilance, to improve standardization and assessment of expectedness and reduce medical judgment subjectivity the use of preferred term (PT) of MedDRA coding is resorted to. If the PT is present in the document it is considered as expected. Otherwise it is considered unexpected.

Minimum Safety Information (MSI)

The minimum information required for expedited reporting purposes is: an identifiable patient, the name of a suspect medicinal product, an identifiable reporting source, and an event.

Information for final description of a case report may not be available for reporting within the regulatory timelines. In such cases initial reports should be submitted as long as the minimum safety criteria are met. Attempts should then be made to obtain relevant, detailed and complete information which can be submitted later as a follow up report.

Expedited Reporting

Serious adverse events and adverse reactions have to be reported on an expedited basis. However there are variations to this dictum. For instance, FDA insists only on serious unexpected reports to be submitted.

Expedited reporting is also indicated in the following scenarios:

- Lack of efficacy of medicinal products used for the treatment of life-threatening diseases, vaccines and contraceptives.

- Any suspected transmission via a medicinal product of an infectious agent is also considered a serious adverse reaction and therefore has to be reported in an expedited manner.

Expedited reporting has to be done if the criteria for expedited reporting is met even if the medicinal product was not used as per guidelines for therapeutic usage as per the SmPC.

The purpose of expedited reporting is to make regulators and other stakeholders aware particularly of new, important information and serious reports. This in turn allows for quicker regulatory decisions.

4. TYPES OF REPORTS

Spontaneous Reports: Health professionals and consumers report adverse events to drugs (including vaccines, X-ray contrast media, traditional and herbal remedies).

Patient's themselves report adverse events after use of a medicine. The patient's relatives such as husband, wife, siblings, or parent can also report any untoward events that the patient is going through after using a medicine. Such reporters are termed Consumers.

Professionals in the healthcare domain such as doctors, dentists, pharmacists, and nurses send reports of events that have occurred in the clinic or hospital or that have been have been reported to them. Such reporters are called healthcare professionals (HCP).

Literature: A sponsor has a literature search team that searches scientific journals and publications and reports events that have been documented wherein their drug is a suspect drug. These are called literature reports

Report from study: The sponsor has to conduct trial of new drugs to obtain approval of the drug as well as observation studies in the post-marketing phase. Adverse events occurring during interventional and noninterventional studies (NIS) or observational studies need to be reported. Such reports are called study reports (report from study). Investigators are responsible for sending reports from study.

5. REPORTING PROCESS

Whom To Report

Adverse events should be reported to the sponsor (company) or to the national regulatory authority.

What Will Happen To The Report?

The report will be submitted to the regulatory adverse event database and will be analyzed by experts.

The database may identity previously unknown, unexpected adverse events or reveal that there is a sudden increase in frequency of some adverse events, or that some patients are more prone to certain adverse events. This can lead to changes in the marketing authorization such as restrictions in use or need for specific warnings in the package insert. When an adverse event is considered totally hazardous, the regulator may order a medicinal product to be withdrawn from the market, which happens only on rare occasions.

During clinical trials, significant adverse events, if suspected to be related to the investigational drug (adverse drug reactions), can lead to changes in the way the medicinal product is developed such as change in dose, dosage regimen, population, and changes to informed consent forms.

The information obtained from the adverse event reports promotes the safe use of medicines on a local, national level and global level.

Focused Studies
Educational And Awareness Programs
Product Package Insert To Include The Possibility Of The Adverse Reaction
Product Package Insert Warnings Such As The Black Box Warning
Changes In The Process Of Manufacture Of The Medicine
Restriction Of Use In Certain Population (Pediatric, Pregnant Women, Geriatric)
Suspension Of Marketing Or Even Withdrawal Of The Product

With growing government and public concern over drug safety, pharmacovigilance (PV) has never been more important. To ensure patient safety, minimize costs and ensure regulatory compliance, sponsors are required to detect and manage drug related risks.

6. SPONTANEOUS REPORTS

Spontaneous reporting is a significant source of global pharmacovigilance reports. Spontaneous reports are submitted voluntarily by healthcare professionals and consumers who identify and report events to their national pharmacovigilance center or to the manufacturer. Spontaneous reporting can happen as an anecdotal report or can be sent via mail, fax, email, can be narrated over the phone, or submitted at websites.

Spontaneous reporting is important for gathering the safety information required for early signal detection. The data collected from spontaneous reports can also be used for conducting risk-benefit analysis of new drugs.

Example Of Spontaneous Reporting: Singapore Regulatory Authority

The Singapore regulatory authority has facilitated submission of spontaneous reports and has given various options to the healthcare professionals and consumers as follows:

Forms may be submitted by mail or fax to Vigilance Branch
Health Products Regulation Group
11 Biopolis Way , #11-03 Helios
Singapore 138667
Fax: (65) 6478 9069
Phone us at Tel: (65) 6866 3538
Email the report to HSA_productsafety@hsa.gov.sg

Adverse events can be reported to the sponsor (company) or to the national regulatory authority- Singapore Regulatory Authority.

What Happens Once A Report Is Submitted To A Sponsor

The sponsor processes the report and submits it to the Singapore regulatory authority within specified timelines.

What Happens Once A Report Is Submitted To The Singapore Regulatory Authority

All the adverse event reporting forms are reviewed, processed and databased by the vigilance department.

Cases can be retrieved from the database according to suspect drugs and adverse events. This information is used in aggregate analysis and aggregate reporting.

Being a member of the WHO International Drug Monitoring Programme, the Singapore regulatory authority then submits these reports to the world bank of adverse events - Uppsala Monitoring Centre in Sweden.

Example Of Spontaneous Reporting: Spontaneous Reporting In USA

FDA receives spontaneous reports from sponsors, hospitals and clinics, healthcare professionals and consumers. Healthcare professionals and consumers report serious adverse events through the FDA Medical Products Reporting Program called MEDWATCH. They can also report directly to the sponsor if they want to.

MEDWATCH reporting can be done by:
Phone (a toll-free number)
Fax
Mail (using a postage-paid form)
Internet (via the interactive form on the MEDWATCH website).

Form FDA 3500 is for voluntary reporting by healthcare professionals, consumers, and patients. The form is to be sent by postage-paid mail or by fax.

Form FDA 3500A is for mandatory reporting by sponsors, distributors, and importers.

Form FDA 3500B is for consumer voluntary reporting.

Report Through MedWatch:

Adverse Events

Patient has undesirable events after taking a drug or using a medical device. Adverse events (new or worsening of pre- existing symptoms) after taking a drug or using a device can be reported using a Medwatch form.

Medication Error

Any medication error such as drug misuse, abuse, overdose, inappropriate schedule of drug administration, or instances of wrong drug administered or similar label appearance that could possibly lead to error regardless of patient involvement and outcome. If a drug or device is not used as prescribed or in a manner that could have or has led to unsafe use, then this can be reported using a Medwatch form.

Product Quality Complaint (PQC)

Issues related to the quality, authenticity, performance, or safety of any medication or device can be reported using a Medwatch form.

Different Brand

Differences observed in therapeutic benefit after changing a drug from one brand to a different including loss of efficacy (LOE) can be reported using a Medwatch form.

Do Not Report Through MedWatch:

- Vaccines - Adverse events after vaccination have to be reported to the Vaccine Adverse Event Reporting System (VAERS) at https://vaers.hhs.gov/esub/step1

- Investigational drugs and medical devices - Investigational drug or investigational medical devices adverse events have to be sent to the address of the contact person listed in the study protocol.

FDA Adverse Event Reporting System (FAERS)

The FDA Adverse Event Reporting System (FAERS) is a database that contains information on adverse event and medication error reports submitted to FDA. It is an adverse event database for drugs and therapeutic biological products.

The FDA evaluates spontaneous reporting data from FAERS to identify any serious, rare, or unexpected adverse events or an increased incidence of events.

Drug safety evaluators, product reviewers, medics, and epidemiologists analyze the collected information. Based on the review, further action is decided.

These actions include:

A) Focused studies using epidemiological and analytical databases.

B) After considering the input from these studies, regulatory action may be taken or risk management information may be disseminated including Dear Healthcare Professional letters.

7. TIME FRAMES FOR REGULATORY REPORTING

1. Fatal or Life-Threatening - Fatal or life-threatening clinical trial reports need to be submitted within 7 calendar days after the last received date (day 0).

   Fatal or life-threatening reports where the medicinal product, indication, formulation, or population is not approved may lead to restrictions to the conduct of the trial, including possible suspension of the clinical trial. Hence it is important to submit such reports within the early timeframe.

2. All Other Serious - All other serious adverse reports including spontaneous fatal or life-threatening clinical trial reports must be reported within 15 calendar days after being first received by the sponsor (day 0).

8. CIOMS FORM

- The CIOMS-I form is a standard format for expedited adverse event reporting. It consists of both tabular and narrative presentation of safety data.

- Patient's details and demographics (Name or Initials, identification number, gender, age, height, weight, ethnicity)

- Reporter's details (Name, qualification, profession, place of practice, contact number and email address)

- Details of adverse event (Date of onset , duration, course, therapy and outcome of the event)

- Seriousness criteria

- Suspect drug/s (Brand name, generic, dose, frequency, duration, indication, batch number, expiry date)
- Action taken with suspect drugs including dechallenge and rechallenge

- Concomitant medicines and past drug history

- Medical history

- Relevant information such as allergies, drug allergies, pregnancy, smoking, alcohol and caffeine use or abuse.

Suspect drugs - There can be one or more suspect drugs.
Concomitant medicines – Medicines that are continued to betaken within one month of onset of event.
Past Drugs – Medicines which were taken but stopped on a date which is more than one month of onset of first event.
NKA – No Known Allergy. Report from study - Name of the subject is not used as it is confidential. Instead initials and patient identification number, site/center number and randomization number are used.

CIOMS FORM

CIOMS-I, the WHO International Drug Monitoring Centre (IDMC), and regulatory authorities have laid down the format, information and details that are required for reporting adverse events that occur after taking the suspect drug.

CIOMS

1. Patient Details
   Initials
   Gender
   Age and date of birth
   Weight
   Height

   Other relevant identifier (clinical investigation number, site number, randomization number in case of report from study)

2. Suspect Drug
   Brand name as reported
   International Non-Proprietary Name (INN)
   Batch number
   Indication for which the drug was prescribed or tested
   Dosage form
   Daily dose and regimen (specify units: mg, ml, mg/kg)
   Route of administration
   Start and stop date
   Duration of treatment

   In case of report from study other details such as whether it is in open label or blinded, pretreatment or during treatment is stated.

3. Medical history including allergy, drug or alcohol abuse and family history.

4. Concomitant medications & past drug therapy: The same information as the suspect drug should be provided.

---

5. Details of Adverse Events

Description of the events including anatomical site of occurrence, severity, presentation, signs and symptoms, as well as a diagnosis if available. The seriousness criteria should be indicated.

Start date of onset of reaction

Stop date and duration of reaction

Dechallenge and rechallenge information

Place where the event occurred (e.g., hospital, out-patient clinic, home, nursing home)

Outcome of the events: Information on recovery and any complications or sequelae, laboratory data including test results and reference range. Special investigations and their results.

Treatment of the events including names of medications and procedures with details. Outcome of the events. In case of a fatal outcome, cause of death and a comment on its possible relationship to the suspected reaction should be provided. Details of autopsy findings.

Causality: The reporter may indicate causality such as – related, highly probably related, possibly related, unlikely related and not related.

6. Reporter Information
   Name
   Address
   Telephone number
   Profession (specialty)

7. Administrative Details
Source of report: Was it spontaneous, from a clinical trial interventional, non-interventional or registry, from the literature (literature article to be provided) or other?

Date when report was first received by sponsor
Country in which event occurred

Type of report filed to authorities: initial or follow-up and number of follow up.

Name and address of sponsor
Name, address, telephone number, and FAX number of the reporter

Identifying regulatory code or number for marketing authorization dossier or clinical investigation process for the suspected product (for example IND or CTX number, NDA number)

Sponsor's identification number for the case (this number must be the same for the initial and follow-up reports on the same case).

9. MedDRA

MedDRA: The Medical Dictionary for Regulatory Activities.

MedDRA provides standardized medical terminology. It is developed by ICH (international conference of harmonization). This standardization allows seamless sharing of regulatory information globally for medical products. It is used for registration, documentation and safety monitoring of investigational as well as approved drugs.

MedDRA is meant for coding of events, indications for drug use and medical history.

MedDRA can code for symptoms - dizziness, headache, asthenia; diagnosis- transient Ischemic attack, influenza, multiple sclerosis; syndromes- Steven Johnson Syndrome, Fanconi syndrome, Sjogren syndrome and investigation result - hyponatremia, thrombocytopenia, neutropenia.

The MedDRA dictionary is organized by System Organ Class (SOC), which is divided into High-Level Group Terms (HLGT), High-Level Terms (HLT), Preferred Terms (PT) and finally into Lower-Level Terms (LLT).

The MSSO (Maintenance and Support Services Organization), is contracted by ICH to maintain, develop and distribute Medra. Medra usage is free for regulators, health care providers and academics. However license to use MedDRA is granted to companies only on a paidsubscriptions basis. This payment is calculated taking into account the annual turnover of companies.

Under the governance of the ICH Medra Management Board, MedDRA is updated to meet the needs of regulatory authority and keep up with advances in medical science.

MedDRA has transitioned from version 1 to version 16.0 and currently the LLT has more than sixty thousand terms. This gives more options for each code so that the coder can choose the most appropriate option.

To facilitate its correct use, free training is offered and MedDRA is also made available in several languages - Chinese, Czech, Dutch, French, German, Hungarian, Italian, Japanese, Portuguese and Spanish.

The current ICH M1 Points to Consider Working Group develops and maintains two documents on the use of MedDRA

A.   Data entry

B.   Data retrieval.

The data entry document is for coding purpose and the data retrieval document aids analysis.

The data retrieval document includes guidance on the use of Standardised Medra Queries (SMQs). The SMQ is an efficient tool used in assessment of safety signal detection. Both, the coding as well as the data retrieval documents are generally updated twice a year, and with every MedDRA release.

Collaboration between ICH and WHO: MedDRA is fully implemented in the WHO global safety database allowing entry and retrieval of information not only through WHO-ART but also through MedDRA.

Relationship Between LLT and PT.

PT	A single medical concept.
LLT	A sub-type, lexican variant or synonym of a preferred term.

1. Sub-type: The LLT can be a sub-type of the PT.
   PT   - Limb paresis
   LLT   - Transient paresis of limb
   Here the LLT is more specific and describes the paresis as transient.

   PT   - Influenza
   LLT   - Influenza B virus infection
   Here the LLT describes the type of influenza virus.

   The LLT may specify the anatomical site of the event (ex: generalized), the type of the infection (B virus) or the nature of the event (ex: transient). In the subtype the LLT has more details than the PT.

2. Lexical variants: The terms in the LLT and PT vary. The variation is due to jumbling of word order in and use of abbreviations in the LLT.

A. Jumbled Word order
   PT   - Blood pressure increased
   LLT   - Pressure blood increased

B. Abbreviations
   PT   - Complete Blood Count
   LLT   - CBC

3. Synonyms: Different terms for the same disease. PT is a technical (medical) term.

   PT   - Asthma
   LLT   - Asthma like condition

   PT   - Angina pectoris
   LLT   - Chest pain-cardiac

Example of Event Coding

Example 1.
I have been taking the suspect drug since 3 years. Since six months I have been admitted to the hospital for Crohn' flare.

Search Input : Crohn's
Options that could appear in the MedDRA dictionary :

Crohn's disease
Crohn's aggravated

The appropriate code in this case would be Crohn's aggravated.

Click on the option and the event will be coded to the appropriate PT, HLT, HLGT and SOC.

Reported verbatim: Crohn's flare
Coded to: Crohn's aggravated.

Example 2.
I was on the suspect drug since middle of May in 2005. In December 2009 I was diagnosed with Diabetes Mellitus.

Search Input: Diabetes Mellitus
The options that may appear in the MedDRA dictionary may include:

Type 1 Diabetes Mellitus
Type 2 Diabetes Mellitus
Diabetes Mellitus
Juvenile Diabetes Mellitus

The appropriate option in this case would be Diabetes Mellitus. We cannot choose type 1 or 2 since it is not specified in the source document whether it is type 1 or 2.

In this case you can also choose the autocode option.

The autocode option can be used when the reported terms are highly specific such as dizziness, malaise, hypertension, asthma, Diabetes Mellitus, Parkinson's disease etc.

When you have terms such as weakness of limbs associated with fatigue it is not possible to autocode the reported verbatim. The reported verbatim in this case is: weakness of limbs associated with fatigue.

In case you are not sure or the term does not get autocoded you can choose the manual (interactive) coding option which will throw up a list of options and you will have to choose the most appropriate option.

Example 3

I was on the suspect drug for just a few weeks when I started experiencing pain in the eye and upper limb.

The reported event is: Pain in the eye and upper limb.

In such a scenario it is better to split the term to Pain in the eye Pain in the upper limb.

This can then be coded to Orbital pain Upper limb pain

Example 4

A couple of days after taking the suspect drug my cousin had nausea, vomiting, and abdominal pain. The physician diagnosed gastroenteritis.

This is just the opposite of the earlier example. Here we can just code to gastroenteritis since nausea, vomiting, abdominal pain are known symptoms of gastroenteritis.

Example 5

SOC
Blood and Lymphatic System Disorders

HLGT
White Blood Cell Disorders

HLT
Neutropenias

PT
Neutropenia

LLT
Neutropenia / Neutropenia aggravated

Example 6

SOC
Renal and Urinary disorders

HLGT
Urolithiasis

HLT
Urinary Tract Lithiasis (excl renal)

PT
Calculus Urinary

LLT
Calculus urinary

SYSTEM ORGAN CLASSES

1. Blood and lymphatic system disorders
2. Cardiac disorders
3. Congenital, familial and genetic disorders
4. Labyrinth disorders
5. Musculoskeletal and connective tissue disorders
6. Neoplasms benign, malignant and unspecified (incl cysts and polyps)
7. Endocrine disorders
8. Eye disorders
9. Gastrointestinal disorders
10. Nervous system disorders
11. Pregnancy, puerperium and perinatal conditions
12. General disorders and administration site conditions
13. Hepatobiliary disorders
14. Psychiatric disorders
15. Renal and urinary disorders
16. Reproductive system and breast disorders
17. Immune system disorders
18. Respiratory, thoracic and mediastinal disorders
19. Infections and infestations
20. Injury, poisoning and procedural complications
21. Skin and subcutaneous tissue disorders
22. Social circumstances
23. Surgical and medical procedures
24. Investigations
25. Metabolism and nutrition disorders
26. Vascular disorders

MedDRA Hierarchy (Version 16.1)
System Organ Class (SOC) (26)
High Level Group Term (HLGT) (334)
High Level Term (HLT) (1,717)
Preferred Term (PT) (20,057)
Lowest Level Term (LLT) 71,326

---

10. MedDRA CODING: A PERSPECTIVE

Lowest Level Term that most accurately reflects the reported verbatim information should be selected.

Be specific.

Avoid soft coding.

For lab test results take into consideration absence or presence of units.

Select terms for device-related events, product quality issues, medication errors, medical and social history, investigations and indications. There are many options available to code to the accurate term. Use the search option and familiarize yourselves with the different terms available.

If there is no exact match in MedDRA, use medical judgment to match an existing term (closest possible match) that adequately represents the reported verbatim.

If diagnosis is reported alongwith the signs and symptoms, the preferred option is to code for diagnosis only.

FINAL DIAGNOSIS

Diagnosis along with its characteristic signs symptoms is provided.

Preferred Coding: Diagnosis only.

Example: Pneumonia with fever and cough.

Preferred Coding: Pneumonia.

This is because we know that fever and cough are symptoms of pneumonia.

PROVISIONAL DIAGNOSIS

Provisional diagnosis along with signs and symptoms is provided.

Preferred Coding: Provisional diagnosis plus the signs and symptoms have to be coded.

Example: Possibly a drug allergy with dyspnea and low blood pressure

Preferred Coding: Drug allergy
                   Dyspnea
                   Low blood pressure

SYMPTOMS ONLY

Only symptoms are provided.
Preferred Coding: Code all the reported symptoms.

Example: The patient had fever and cough. Diagnosis was pending
Preferred Coding: Fever
                  Cough

BE SPECIFIC

Being specific is important.

Example: The patient had - paresis of upper limb
Code To: Upper limb paresis and not just to paresis

Example: Stress due to work
Code To: Stress at work and not just to Stress

Use the search option in MedDRA to select the most specific code.

AVOID SOFT CODING

Coding to a less severe medical condition is termed as soft coding. This has to be avoided.

Example: "End stage renal failure" coded as "Renal impairment"

While there is renal impairment it does not convey that the patient has progressed to end stage renal failure. An inappropriate coding is a wrong coding.

COMBINATION TERMS

Use combination terms whenever available.

Example: Cardiomyopathy due to diabetes
Code To: Diabetic cardiomyopathy

SPLIT TERMS

Split terms when it describes two possible codes.
Example: Pruritic generalized rash
Code To: Generalized rash
           Pruritic rash

LACK OF EFFICACY (LOE)

Example: The drug did not work
Code To: Lack of drug effect

Example: Patient took the drug for several weeks. Now the drug is not working as it used to.
Code To: Drug effect decreased

UNCLEAR TERMINOLOGY

The source document has thin details and no clarity.

Example: Became pink
Code to: Unevaluable event

"Bacame pink" is vague. It could be that the patient became pink, skin turned pink, possibly an erythema or the syrup color turned pink. Some symptom has been reported but when it could mean so many possibilities it becomes an unevaluable event.

Example: Patient had a problem with his liver
Code To: Liver disorder

Example: Patient had a medical condition and went for investigations
Code To: Ill-defined disorder

This is a general statement. Possibly the reporter had only this information at the time of reporting.

MEDICATION ERRORS

Example: Last week the patient missed taking a dose
Code To: Drug dose omission

Example: Patient received an overdose of medicine
Code To: Drug overdose

Example: Patient with G6PD deficiency is prescribed a drug that is contraindicated in this condition.
Code To: Labeled drug-disease interaction medication error.

These are medication errors without any associated events. So just code to the reported verbatim.

MEDICATION ERRORS WITH ADVERSE EVENTS

Example: Patient was administered wrong drug and experienced dyspnea
Code To: Wrong drug administered
        Dyspnea

Example: Because of similar sounding drug names, the patient took the wrong drug and developed oedema
Code To: Drug name confusion
          Wrong drug administered
          Oedema

Example: There was a prescription error and the patient had diplopia
Code To: Drug prescribing error
          Diplopia

Prescription errors – When doctor's do not follow the recommendations and cross the maximum or minimum dose or frequency when prescribing a drug.

The other prescription errors are:

Drug dose prescribing error
Drug dosage form prescribing error
Drug dose schedule prescribing error
Drug route prescribing error

As you can see in addition to the events that have occurred it is also mandatory to capture and code the associated medication errors. Note that there are various types of medication errors and these have to be identified and coded appropriately.

INVESTIGATION RESULT CODING

Example: Hb 8 g/dl
Code To: Haemoglobin low

Units are given and so we can be sure that the result is low

Example: Calcium 3.3
Code To: Blood calcium abnormal

The calcium normal values are 8.5 to 10.5 mg/dL and also 2.12 to 2.62 mmol/L.

This could be high or low calcium depending on the units. Since units are not provided code to calcium abnormal.

11. ACTION TAKEN, DC AND RC

Scenario 1.

1. The patient is taking the suspect drug for cataplexy and narcolepsy since 5 weeks after which she has recurring episodes of migraine. She consults her physician who advises her to discontinue the suspect drug. The patient discontinues the suspect drug. Six months later the episodes of migraine resolve. The patient restarts the suspect drug. Two months later the migraine episodes reappear.

Action taken - Drug withdrawn
Dechallenge - Positive
Rechallenge - Positive

On drug withdrawal the adverse event resolves.
Dechallenge - Positive

On reintroduction of the suspect drug the adverse event reappears.
Rechallenge - Positive

Rechallege is possible only when dechallenge is positive.

Scenario 2

The patient was on the suspect drug since 2 years for rheumatoid arthritis. Recently investigations revealed a high level of liver function tests. Suspect drug was suspended. After a gap of a few days the suspect drug was reintroduced. The liver function tests were drastically high.

Action taken - Drug withdrawn
Dechallenge - Unknown
Rechallenge - Not Applicable

Suspect drug was suspended.
Action taken - Drug withdrawn

Outcome of the event high level of liver function tests is not given.
Dechallenge – Unknown
Rechallenge comes into play only when dechallenge is positive.
Rechallenge - Not Applicable

Scenario 3

The patient was on the suspect drug for allergic rhinitis. The allergic rhinitis resolved and the suspect drug was discontinued. A couple of days later the patient had pyrexia.

Action taken - Not applicable
Dechallenge - Not applicable
Rechallenge - Not applicable.

When the suspect drug is discontinued prior to onset of the adverse event the action taken is not applicable.

Scenario 4

The patient was on the suspect drug for nine years. Last year he was diagnosed with astrocytoma. The suspect drug was discontinued. The astrocytoma was ongoing and the patient was scheduled for consultation with the neurosurgeon for management of the brain tumour.

Action Taken - Drug withdrawn
Dechallenge - Negative
Rechallenge - Not applicable

The suspect drug was not restarted. Hence rechallenge is not applicable.

Scenario 5

The patient was on the suspect drug for primary hypertension. The patient reported feeling weak. On examination he had pedal edema. The suspect drug was withdrawn. The events did not resolve. The suspect drug was restarted.

Action Taken - Drug withdrawn
Dechallenge - Negative
Rechallenge - Not applicable

When the adverse event is ongoing even after drug withdrawal, dechallenge is negative. When dechallenge is negative rechallenge is not applicable.

Rechallege is possible only when dechallenge is positive. In this case dechallenge is negative hence there is no question of rechallenge.

Scenario 6

The patient was on the suspect drug for middle insomnia. After being on the suspect drug for a week she reported vertigo and hyperhidrosis. The suspect drug was continued.

Action taken - Dose not changed
Dechallenge - Not applicable
Rechallenge - Not applicable

Dechallenge happens only when the drug is withdrawn or dose of the suspect drug is reduced. In this case the drug is continued. Hence dechallenge is not applicable.

Scenario 7

The patient was on the suspect drug and developed hypoesthesia over the left arm. The dose of the suspect drug was reduced. The hypoesthesia improved.

Action taken - Dose reduced
Dechallenge - Positive

The event hypoesthesia improved on dechallenge.

Action taken can be the following:

Dose not changed

Dose increased

Dose reduced

Drug withdrawn

Not applicable

Unknown

Dechallenge can be initiated either by dose reduction or drug withdrawal.

12. WHO DRUG DICTIONARY

The WHO Drug Dictionary (WHO DD) is a classification of medicines by the WHO Program for International Drug Monitoring. It is managed by the Uppsala Monitoring Centre (UMC).

It is used by sponsors, clinical research organizations and regulatory authorities for identification and coding of drugs in spontaneous and clinical trial reports.

The new WHO Drug Dictionary Enhanced is the result of collaboration of UMC with IMS Health. It contains data from the WHO Drug Dictionary and also from IMS Health and has been developed using formats which are similar to those in the WHO Drug Dictionary.

The WHO Drug Dictionary Enhanced contains the most number of product names and is the most comprehensive drug product information. Many suspect, concomitant or past drugs can easily have a direct match and this in turn can lead to increased accuracy and speed of drug coding.

Brand drugs need to be input and coded to its generic using the WHO DD. Generics have to coded as reported.

13. CAUSALITY ASSESSMENT

Causality refers to the cause of the adverse events. Causality assessment tries to examine whether the suspect drug itself was the cause of the adverse events that occur after starting the drug.

Causality assessment is required for clinical trial cases. However, spontaneous reports usually imply causality. For purposes of reporting, spontaneous cases are considered as related by default.

Terms that describe the degree of causality between a drug and an event are - certain, definitely, highly probable, probably, possibly, and likely related. Phrases such as "plausible relationship," "suspected causality," "causal relationship cannot be ruled out" and "reasonable causal relationship are also used to describe the various degrees of causal relationship.

Global Introspection

The global introspection method of causality assessment refers to causality assessment done by experienced physicians. Therefore the outcome depends on the proficiency, expertise and judgment of the physicians.

The causality assessor uses information regarding dechallenge, rechallenge, lack of alternative factors, known class effect and co-factors such as concomitant medication and medical history while evaluating the causality. Inspite of evaluating the causality based on such criteria this method of causality assessment has been termed as being subjective.

Algorithm

Algorithms when used alone may not be accurate as they may not be the alternative to global introspection.
However this method too has its uses.

Algorithm based causality scales:

- WHO assessment scale
- Karch and Lasagna's scale
- Kramer scale
- Yale logarithm
- European ABO system.

A commonly used algorithm based causality scale is the Naranjo ADR probability scale designed by Naranjo.

It has a questionnaire to which scores are allotted. Depending on the final total score the causality is defined as being definite, probable, possible or doubtful.

Resolution of the event when the suspect drug is withdrawn is a strong possibility of the drug being the cause of the symptom.

Latency refers to time to onset (The duration between start of the suspect drug and the start of the event). Dechallenge means withdrawal of drug or drug dose reduction.

Positive dechallenge happens when there is improvement or complete recovery on dechallenge.

Negative dechallenge happens when the event isongoing even after dechallenge.

Rechallenge means reintroducing the drug after a positive dechallenge.

In reports of clinical trials the terms used are– related, probably related, possibly related, unlikely related and not related.

As per FDA a separate causality assessment has to be done for study cases – Investigator's (reporter's) causality and company (sponsor's) causality.

If there is difference between 2 assessments of causality the worst case scenario must be reported. For instance if 2 independent assessments are done and state Related and Not Related, then the causality would be Related. The EMEA states that if there is difference between the sponsor and the investigator's causality the sponsor cannot downgrade the investigator's causality.

Question	Yes	No	Do Not Know	Score
1. Are there previous conclusive reports on this reaction	+1	0	0	
2. Did the adverse event appear after the suspect drug was administered	+2	-1	0	
3. Did the adverse event abate (improve) when the suspect drug was withdrawn	+1	0	0	
4. Did the adverse event reappear when the drug was re-administered	-1	+2	0	
5. Are there alternative causes or factors that could on their own have caused the reaction	-1	+1	0	
6. Did the reaction reappear when a placebo was administered	+1	0	0	
7. Was the drug detected in blood or other body fluids in toxic concentrations	+1	0	0	
8. Was the reaction more severe when the dose was increased or less severe when the dose was decreased	+1	0	0	
9. Did the patient have a similar reaction to the same or similar drugs in any previous exposure	+1	0	0	
10. Was the adverse event confirmed by any objective evidence (such as lab tests)	+1	0	0	
Total Score:				

Total Score

- > 9: definite
- 5-8: probable
- 1-4:possible
- 0   :doubtful

14. UNBLINDING & SUSAR

Blinding and randomization are required for avoiding both investigator as well as subject bias.

Inappropriate unblinding may lead to investigator or subject bias. Subject may misinterpret the unblinded results and may further spread misinformation regarding efficacy and toxicity to other subjects.

Unblinding

In a double blind study the investigator and the subjects are not aware whether they are on the investigational drug or the comparator - placebo or active comparator. In a double blind study when the causality of a serious event is considered to be related and the event is unexpected as per the investigator's brochure (IB) then this results in a SUSAR (serious unexpected suspected adverse reaction). However prior to submitting a SUSAR report to the regulatory authorities such cases require unblinding. The blind is broken only for that particular subject.

The site number, randomization number, subject numbers are sent to the sponsor appointed physician in charge of unblinding. These numbers help the physician identify the subject accurately. The physician then unblinds case.

Once the blind is broken it is known whether the subject was on the investigational drug, the placebo or the active comparator. This makes it clear whether the sponsor's investigational drug was responsible for the SUSAR or it was the placebo or active comparator.

The SUSAR is ticked Yes - Pla/comp when the subject after unblinding is found to be on either placebo (if the therapeutic physician considers the excipient to be a factor) or the active comparator (standard drug) and the event that has occurred is considered unexpected.

The SUSAR is ticked YES – (company drug) when the subject after unblinding is found to be on the investigational new drug (sponsor drug) and the event is unexpected as per the IB.

SUSAR is generated only for report from study and not for spontaneous reports.

15. POST STUDY & PRE TREATMENT CASES

Active Comparator

The sponsor can decide whether active comparator drug reactions should be reported to the other manufacturer and/or directly to the appropriate regulatory agencies.

Post-study Cases

Serious adverse events that take place after the patient has completed a clinical study (including any protocol required post-treatment follow-up) will possibly be reported by an investigator to the sponsor. Such cases should be regarded for expedited reporting purposes as though they were study reports.

Pre-Treatment Cases

Events which occur even before the investigational drug is administered are termed as pre-treatment cases. In such cases the subject would have entered the study by signing the informed consent form. But the subject would not have started receiving the investigational drug. Pretreatment cases are not submitted to the regulatory authority but only data based with the sponsor.

16. WORKFLOW

Reports

Spontaneous (consumer, HCP), Literature, Report from study (Investigator)

Identify & Segregate Serious from Non-Serious report.

Serious	Non-Serious
Case Processing	Case Processing
Narrative Writing	Narrative Writing
Case Review	Case Review
Case Approval	Case Approval

Case Processing

Adverse events, medical history and indication for the suspect drug are identified, lab tests are input and all these are coded using MeDdra.

Suspect drug, concomitant medication and past drugs are identified and coded using the WHO DD.

Information regarding the LRD, affiliate ID, patient demographics are also input.

Narrative Writing

Narratives are written as per format.

Case Review

Expectedness of the events is assessed, company causality is input for report from studies, SUSAR is ticked
–Yes or No for report from study cases.

Case Approval

The case is then approved to be submitted to the regulatory authority.

17. THE PHARMACOVIGILANCE SYSTEM

A pharmacovigilance system is designed to monitor the safety of medicines and to detect any change to their risk-benefit profile. In addition, it enables an organization to carry out its legal responsibilities with regards to pharmacovigilance. An ideal pharmacovigilance system should be well structured and have processes aligned to outcomes. EMEA (European Medicines Evaluation Agency) has emerged as a global leader in pioneering pharmacovigilance systems and has created a state of art pharmacovigilance system called Eudravigilance.

An ideal system is never static but undergoes changes to incorporate current standards.

EUDRAVIGILANCE

EudraVigilance is a data processing network and management system for reporting and assessment of suspected adverse reactions that occur during the development and post the marketing authorization of medicinal products in the European Economic Area (EEA). The first operating version was launched in December 2001. Eudravigilance is at the core of the European Risk Management Strategy, initiated by EMEA and the national regulatory authorities. The objective of Eudravigilance is to streamline the process of risk management which includes risk detection, risk assessment, risk minimisation and risk communication.

EudraVigilance

- lElectronic exchange of Individual Case Safety Reports (ICSR's) between the European Medicines Evaluation Agency (EMEA), national regulatory

- authorities, marketing authorization holders, and sponsors of clinical trials in the EEA.

- lEarly detection of potential safety signals.

- lContinuous monitoring of safety parameters.

- lData based decision making process of the drug safety profile.

- lRisk Management.

EudraVigilance provides two reporting modules:

1. EudraVigilance Clinical Trial Module: For ICSR's that need to be reported during clinical trials in the pre approval phase.

2. EudraVigilance Post-Marketing Module: For ICSR's that need to be reported in the post marketing phase.

Eudravigilance contributes to the promotion of the individual patient and the public health in the EEA and is an efficient system for the EMEA and national regulatory authorities to regulate drug safety.

European Medicines Evaluation Agency (EMEA). The EMEA is the centralized regulatory authority for the European Union (EU).

Volume 9 of 'The rules governing medicinal products in the European Union (Eudralex)' was prepared by the European Commission in consultation with EMEA, states of the EEA and stakeholders. It provides guidance for the marketing authorization holders and national regulatory authorities regarding the requirements, procedures, roles and activities related to pharmacovigilance. This guidance is for both human and veterinary medicinal products and also incorporates the International Conference on Harmonisation (ICH) and the Veterinary International Conference on Harmonisation (VICH) guidelines.

Volume 9 has four parts:

Part I - Pharmacovigilance of medicinal products for human use.

Part II - Pharmacovigilance of veterinary medicinal products.

Part III - General information on EU electronic exchange of pharmacovigilance data.

Part IV - General reference to administrative and legislative

Volume 9A of Eudralex - "Rules Governing Medicinal Products in the European Union: Pharmacovigilance for medicinal products for human use".

18. Good Pharmacovigilance Practice Guidelines (GVP)

The EMEA introduced the new pharmacovigilance legislation from 02 July 2012. With this Volume 9A is replaced by the good pharmacovigilance practice guidelines (GVP) initiated by the EMEA.

A. Proactive risk management is expected from the sponsors
B. Higher quality of safety data
C. Safety assessments lead to immediate regulatory action
D. Clear responsibilities for marketing authorizationholders and the regulatory authorities
E. A new scientific committee at the European Medicines Agency: The Pharmacovigilance Risk Assessment Committee
F. Patient involvement in committee meetings. This is a significant change

The New Pharmacovigilance Legislation Changes

Reporting

- Single window submission. The EMEA now requires centralized reporting. Reports have to be submitted only to EMEA-Eudravigilance and not to each regulatory authority.

Report all serious suspected adverse reactions directly to the EudraVigilance database. Reports concerning compassionate use or named patient should also be submitted to EudraVigilance.

- Adverse drug reaction now refers to all undesirable events that have occurred in a patient that are "noxious and unintended". This means that in addition to events that are occurring at proper dose and dosage regimen, those events that occur due to medication error, misuse, abuse and offlabel cases should also be reported.

Definition of Adverse Reaction

A response to a medicinal product which is noxious and unintended and

Before GVP

which occurs at doses normally used in man

After GVP

Which occurs within or outside the marketing authorization conditions or from occupational exposure.

So now adverse events for reporting to EMEA includes events that occur even after off-label use, overdose, misuse, abuse, medication errors and after occupational exposure.

- Reports from patients are now required to be submitted.

- The new EU pharmacovigilance legislation also introduces mandatory reporting of non-serious suspected adverse drug reactions within a timeline of 90 days.

- MAHs have a responsibility to review websites under their control and report valid cases. They do not have to search sites which are not under their control.

- The E2B (R2) standard is the current reporting format. MAHs will be required to implement the new ICSR E2B (R3) which will come into effect in 2016.

- Under the new legislation specified medicinal products will be authorized subject to additional monitoring due to their safety profile. Those products will be identified with a symbol which shall be selected by the Commission possibly by July 2013.

Marketing Applications

In new applications Detailed Description of the Pharmacovigilance System (DDPS) has been replaced by the Pharmacovigilance System Master File (PSMF). The PSMF won't have to be formally submitted, but it should be made available by the sponsor on request to the regulatory authority.

Initial marketing authorisation (MA) applications after 21-Jul-2012 will be accepted only if they include a Risk Management Plan (RMP).

Renewal applications will no longer require a Periodic Safety Update Report (PSUR). However, the Addendum to the Clinical Overview should now include a benefit-risk evaluation and an updated Risk Management Plan (RMP).

PSUR

The periodic safety update reports are needed for evaluation of the risk-benefit profile of a medicinal product at specified regulatory timelines during the post-authorization phase. This allows for an ongoing assessment of benefit versus risk of the drug.

- The new format is PBRER: ICH - E2C (R2)
- Periodic safety reports may not be routinely required for low risk, generic and well-established drugs.

The PSUR provides an assessment of the drug risk versus benefit after inclusion of the emerging safety data. The format has been revised to incorporate a renewed focus on the safety profile while making it less cumbersome and more efficient. The new format is called PBRER. There will be no routine requirement for line listings

PBRER-Periodic Benefit-Risk Evaluation Report

The main focus of each PBRER is the evaluation of relevant new safety information and conducting an Integrated benefit risk evaluation for approved indications.

The PBRER should include the proposed actions which the MAH intends to undertake to improve the safety profile.

A drug is approved by regulatory authorities only after they are convinced that it has a favorable benefit-risk profile. As post marketing information keeps coming in, evaluation should be continued to find out whether benefits continue to be more than the risks. This evaluation should also suggest risk minimization actions that the MAH can initiate.

The PBRER has a modular format which enables the use of the modules across multiple regulatory documents. This helps improve efficiency by reducing duplication of effort. There will be new evaluation sections to support this approach to integrated analysis, including a section to give an overview on signals.

Pharmacovigilance System Master File (PSMF)
This is the master file and contains details of:
Training
Inspections - Audits
Safety Profile
Risk Management Plans (RMP)
Literature Information
Signal Management
Case Reporting
Legal & Regulatory framework

Signal Management
The MAH should monitor data with an objective of identifying potential safety risks on a continuous basis. The MAH should also monitor the Eudravigilance database as per their access limits. Signals undergo validation, prioritization and assessment. The signal detection quality management system includes an audit trail.

Signal management is carried to identify new risks and also to find out whether known risks have changed.

Based on an examination of individual case safety reports (ICSRs), aggregated data from active surveillance systems or studies, literature information and other sources.
• Signal detection
• Validation
• Prioritization
• In depth assessment to confirm or refute
• Action taken to manage the signal.

Drugs which are under additional monitoring will require more frequent signal detection. MAHs will need to provide the reason why certain drugs are looked at more frequently than others.

Signals are categorized as new, ongoing or closed.

Safety Communication

- Common language and includes print, web communication and responding to concerns and issues that the public has with the drug.
- Direct Healthcare Professional Communication (DHPC)
- Regulatory communication

RMP

Required for all new marketing applications including for new doses, dosage forms, route of administrations and indications.

Additional Monitoring

Drugs requiring additional monitoring by the regulatory authorities have a Black Triangle symbol. HCPs and consumers are educated on how to report for drugs as per the additional monitoring policy.

PRAC

A new committee, the Pharmacovigilance Risk Assessment Committee (PRAC) will support the EMA's scientific advisory committee (CHMP). PRAC began a new assessment procedure for centrally authorized products in 2012. Under this procedure, findings lead to automatic regulatory action -- variation, suspension or revocation.

Public can henceforth attend PRAC meetings of drug safety profiles. This is a significant development in the area of risk communication and awareness.

GVP (Good Pharmacovigilance Practice) MODULES

Module I	Pharmacovigilance systems and their quality systems
Module II	Pharmacovigilance system master file (PSMF)
Module III	Pharmacovigilance inspections
Module IV	Pharmacovigilance audits
Module V	Risk management systems
Module VI	Management and reporting of adverse reactions
Module VII	Periodic safety update report
Module VIII	Post-authorisation safety studies
Module VIII addendum I	Member States' requirements for transmission of information on non-interventional post-authorisation safety studies
Module IX	Signal management
Module X	Additional monitoring
XI	Public participation in pharmacovigilance
XII	Continuous pharmacovigilance, ongoing benefit-risk evaluation, regulatory action and planning of public communication
XIV	International cooperation
Module XV	Safety communication
ModuleXVI	Risk-minimization measures: selection of tools and effectiveness indicators

SERIOUS EEA REPORTS		
	CURRENT	GVP
Health professional	Within15 Days - To national regulatory authority	To EudraVigilance Within 15 Days
Consumer	Submission Not Required	To EudraVigilance Within 15 Days

EEA Consumer reports were currently not being submitted.

OUTSIDE EEA SERIOUS REPORT		
	CURRENT	GVP
Health professional	Within15 Days	To EudraVigilance Within 15 Days
Consumer	Not Required	To EudraVigilance Within 15 Days

Outside EEA Consumer reports were currently not being submitted.

NON SERIOUS EEA REPORTS		
	CURRENT	GVP
Health professional	Submission Not Required	To EudraVigilance Within 90 Days
Consumer	Submission Not Required	To EudraVigilance Within 90 Days

EEA Non-serious reports were currently not being submitted.

OUTSIDE EEA NON SERIOUS REPORT		
	CURRENT	GVP
Health professional	Not Required	Not Required
Consumer	Not Required	Not Required

Outside EEA Non-serious reports were currently not being submitted and will not be required to be submitted.

QPPv

The marketing authorization holder needs to have a qualified person responsible for pharmacovigilance in the European Union. This person should have experience in all aspects of pharmacovigilance and if not medically qualified should have access to a medically qualified person. National regulations in some states require a nominated individual in that country who has specific legal obligations in respect of pharmacovigilance at a national level.

The responsibilities of the qualified person responsible for pharmacovigilance are:

- lEstablishment and maintenance of a system which ensures that information about all adverse events which are reported to the marketing authorization holder, is collected and databased.

- lPreparation of reports- adverse drug reaction (ADR) reports, Periodic Safety Update Reports (PSURs), company sponsored post-authorization study reports.

- lDechallenge and Rechallenge outcomes to be documented.

19. FDA: ADJUDICATION AND ADVISORY PANEL

Adjudication and Advisory Committee Panel are part of the regulatory approval process in the FDA.

FDA Adjudication

The FDA adjudication involves independent assessment by competent and experienced medical specialists of the clinical end points.

Basically, adjudication attempts to conclude whether:

1) The adverse events that occurred in the clinical trials were expected to occur in the populations studied?

2) The events were in any degree related to the study drug?

If they were expected to occur then the causality is weakened to that extent

FDA Advisory Committee Panel

The FDA Advisory Committee Pane consists of several eminent professionals who vote on medical issues and whether to grant approval or not.

For instance, recently an FDA advisory panel - The FDA Endocrinologic and Metabolic Drugs Advisory Committee voted against approval of lorcaserin as a weightloss drug for obese patients by a 9-5 vote.

The FDA is not bound to follow the advice of its advisory committees, but it more often than not goes along with the decision of its advisory committee panel.

20. BACK TO THE FUTURE - MODERN HISTORY

VIOXX

Rofecoxib, a nonsteroidal anti-inflammatory drug was indicated for treatment of pain conditions in arthritic patients. The Food and Drug Administration (FDA) approved Rofecoxib in1999, and it was marketed by Merck under the brand name Vioxx. Vioxx gained widespread acceptance among doctors and an estimated 80 million patients were prescribed rofecoxib through its lifecycle.

But not everything was fine. Clinical trial reports were pointing towards the significant risk of myocardial infarction, stroke and death associated with long-term use of rofecoxib. In 2001, based on the results of the VIGOR study the FDA sent a warning letter to the CEO of Merck, stating that patients on Vioxx were observed to have a four to five fold increase in myocardial infarctions (MIs) compared to patients on the comparator but the marketing campaign by Merck had not addressed this adequately. Subsequent to this observation by the FDA Merck in the year 2002 incorporated labeling warnings concerning the increased risk of heart attack and stroke.

But, it was only in 2004 that Merck decided to withdraw Vioxx from the market. By then Vioxx was believed to have led to about 60,000 deaths.

There was a negotiated settlement between the sponsor and the Justice Department of the United States of America. This was part of a series of fraud cases initiated by federal prosecutors against big pharmaceutical companies.

There has been much debate and there have been questions some of which perhaps did not have convincing answers.

1. Was there effective disclosure and interpretation of trial findings? Why did the sponsor not give due importance to study findings?

2. Was there effective and timely public awareness of safety profile? One of the prime focus of the ERICE declaration.

3. Should the sponsor have taken the warning more seriously rather than just initiating labeling change?

4. Should not the sponsor have initiated more focused studies at an early stage?

5. In view of the life threatening or possibly fatal risk should the regulator have initiated more stringent action?

6. Why did the sponsor or the regulator not consider safety steps such as delaying the drug release, suspension of the drug at least in high risk patients?

SERVIER MEDIATOR

Servier, France's second-largest drugmaker was the manufacturer of Mediator- benfluorex. About 5 million people had consumed Mediator, between 1976 and November 2009.

Mediator was prescribed as an appetite suppressant for diabetic patients.

It was insinuated that Servier's Mediator - benfluorex, was left on the market long after serious medical issues began to emerge. It was withdrawn in France, only several years after it was discontinued in Spain and Italy. Benfluorex, is closely pharmacologically related to fenfluramine (weight loss drug). Fenfluramine itself was withdrawn in the USA in the year 1997 after being associated with heart-valve damage.

Mediator was finally linked to heart-valve damage and the investigators reiterated that the risks were deliberately concealed. The French health ministry stated that at least 500 people died of Mediator related heart-valve disorders. The fatalities could be upto 2,000. Investigations also looked into the process of obtaining authorization and the aspect of dishonest practices involving regulatory officials. This made the Mediator case scandalous and the furor that erupted led to major regulatory changes not only in France and but entire Europe itself.

Was there a scientific validity to Mediato'rs intended role as a diabetic medication? Was there violation of a basic tenet of ICH-GCP – Risk to human life is of paramount concern.

The Mediator case draws attention to whether there was blatant disregard of risk to human life in the pursuit of profits.

As part of pharmacovigilance you will come across not only inadvertent errors or errors in judgment but also willful deception. You will be up against them. But I will leave you with a sterling example which will speak to you much more effectively than anything I can say:

KESLEY & THE THALIDOMIDE DISASTER

A German pharmaceutical company developed thalidomide in the 1950's as a sleeping pill. It was also found to be useful in relieving the symptoms of morning sickness in pregnant women. In 1960, the company applied to the FDA for approval to sell thalidomide in the United States of America.

At that time thalidomide was very popular in Europe. The file for approval was handed over to Ms. Frances Kelsey – a new medical reviewer. The approval was considered to be a cake walk by many experts.

However Frances had other ideas. Frances found it strange that while thalidomide had no reported harmful effects in animals, it also did not have the beneficial effect of making them sleepy. It was apparent to Frances that the effect of the drug in animals was different from that in humans. Moreover it was disconcerting to her that not much was known about its adverse event profile.

The company pressured Frances several times. But she would not approve until she had proof of it being safe.

In 1961, Frances read in the British Medical Journal that long-term use of thalidomide caused tingling, numbness, and burning pain in the fingers and toes. The article also further stated that the cause could be nerve damage.

It was apparent to Frances that a drug that damaged nerves could be harmful to a developing fetus. She began to consider the possibility that thalidomide could have a teratogenic toxicity profile.

It was not much later that reports of various birth defects began to pour in and countries one by one began to ban thalidomide. It was sold from 1957 to 1962 as medication for morning sickness. By then more than 10,000 children in about 46 countries were born with birth deformities such as phocomelia and there were thousands of reported fatalities. The German company withdrew their application for approval in the United States.

In 1962, Frances Kesely was praised by the media as "the heroine who prevented what could have been an appalling American tragedy, the birth of hundreds or indeed thousands of armless and legless children." Kelsey received the highest award for civilian service from President Kennedy. A New York Times article lauded Kelsey for winning "a two-year battle with the makers of thalidomide."

THE FUTURE

Penicillin was an inadvertent discovery in a petri dish and spawned an era of antibiotics. Today, biomolecular engineering has created an entirely new set of drug class - biologics. Biologics includes recombinant proteins such as Erythropoietin (EPO) and Granulocyte colony-stimulating factor (G-CSF), monoclonal antibodies such as Humira (adalumimab), Enbrel (etanercept), Rituxan (rituximab), h uma nizedmonoclonalantibodiessuchas Herceptin(trastuzumab) and stem cell therapy.

Monoclonal antibodies are used to treat cancer, autoimmune and inflammatory diseases. Not something that was so common just a decade back. But these bring another issue for the regulators. With small-molecule drugs, generics are possible. But with biologics, generic manufacturers may not be able to reproduce exact versions. Since biologics are complex molecules regulatory approval of biosimilars is a highly complicated issue. Regulatory approval for biologics does not exist in most countries as of now.

Stem cell research was the latest and we are already talking of individualized therapy based on genetic profile of a person.

All these increse the complex of pharmacovigilance. Pharmacovigilance may need specialists to handle such a diverse portfolio of drugs and drug classes and to keep pace with fast changing medical therapy and advances in biotech and genomic technology.

Expanding use of websites to report events have created another easy avenue of event reporting. Regulatory framework will start pharmacovigilance activity in regions where it was not going on earlier. This will increase the overall size of pharmacovigilance.

Pharmacovigilance will increase in size and complexity. And pharmacovigilance will increase in possibilities.

21. RULES & REGULATIONS

The European Council has approved new European drug safety legislation. The changes were influenced also by the Servier's Mediator – benfluorex scandal.

The new Regulation and Directive on Pharmacovigilance has the following features:

Use of standard black symbol for drugs that require closer monitoring.

Drugs that have market authorization in more than one member state to have an automatic review process at an European Union level, if they carry serious risk issues.

Drugs whose approval depends upon postauthorization safety studies to be in increased monitoring list.

Sponsors to be made more forthcoming, factual and accurate about the reasons for the withdrawal of a drug from the market.

Were the regulations not existing or not enough to have examples such as Vioxx and Mediator.

Or are we as part of pharmacovigilance not enforcing them. Make more laws and regulations if required. But these need to be enforced.

So, as you can see, by being part of pharmacovigilance we can save lives. In thousands. But, we as pharmacovigilance specialists need to act. We have the power to enforce. Enforce.

Frances Kesley

She would not approve until
she had proof of it being safe.

The only rule.

Assessment of Seriousness from Social Media

The child was taking adult dose of the suspect drug and the seizures were well controlled. The child was brought to hospital for vaccination. There the dose was corrected to child dose. On taking the child dose the child had a seizure which was huge.

Assess the seriousness of the case.

Social media reports of adverse events can have more impact to the reader but little by means of essential details on which one can database the case accurately. Some of them can be outright confusing. Hence assessment of social media cases can be a challenge in itself.

22. SIGNAL DETECTION

WHO definition: Reported information on a possible causal relationship between an adverse event and a drug, the relationship being unknown or incompletely documented previously.

The CIOMS Working Group VIII (CIOMS, Geneva 2010) definition: A signal is information that arises from one or multiple sources (including observations and experiments), which suggests a new potentially causal association, or a new aspect of a known association, between an intervention and an event or set of related events, either adverse or beneficial, that is judged to be of sufficient likelihood to justify verificatory action.

Signal detection (SD) is advanced safety surveillance. The objective of signal detection is to identify adverse events that were earlier considered unexpected or were unknown and appropriately highlight this in the labeling information.

Usually more than a single report is required to generate a signal, depending upon the event and quality of the information available.

Signal detection involves a range of techniques. Data mining is an approach in signal detection that has gained importance due to availability of computed programs. Data mining is carried out on the databases that are available with the sponsor or a regulatory authority. Individual Case Safety Reports from such databases are retrieved and converted into structured format. Statistical algorithms are applied to this structured dataset to calculate measures of association. If the statistical measure crosses a set threshold, then it is considered to be a signal. Signals are typically generated in drug-event pairs - an adverse event associated with a particular drug. Signals which are significant require further analysis using all available data either to confirm or refute the signal. If this in-depth analysis is non-conclusive, more data may be needed which can be obtained by initiating specific studies such as a post-marketing observational trial.

The detection of early warning signs has certain challenges:

- Adverse drug effects are heterogenous and require meticulous analysis.
- New signals may differ from earlier signals lending to possible confusion.
- Signals are both qualitative and quantitative and both aspects need to be addressed.
- Different types of adverse events require different methods for detection.
- Signal detection should ultimately inform whether risks have changed.

Types of events

Type A: Events related to the pharmaceutical activity of the drug and are dosage dependent.

Type B: Allergic or unpredictable reactions and mostly not dosage dependent. These are seen in a small subset of patients.

Type C: Events that occur due to a disease rather than as an outcome of drug usage.

Pharmacovigilance is mainly able to detect type B and unusual type A events. Analysis of Type C events is complex and poses a challenge.

PROCESS OF SIGNAL DETECTION

Signals are obtained by analysis of reports from spontaneous reports, prescription event monitoring, case-control surveillance, literature information, registries and studies - clinical trials or non-interventional studies.

Signals from spontaneous reports may be detected from ICSRs, literature, PBRERs and information from regulatory documents such as variations, renewals, and risk-benefit plans. Poison centers, teratology information services or vaccine surveillance programs also contribute ICSRs in addition to reports from consumers and HCPs.

Active surveillance is based on coordination with healthcare professionals for prescription event monitoring. Creating a network of general practitioners and clinics allows reporting of specified events or events for specified drugs. Signals may arise from studies - interventional and observational, meta-analyses, registries (AED – antiepileptic drug registry, pregnancy registry etc) and literature search.

Strength of evidence in a signal depends on the following factors: Strength of the association: Are there associated causative factors other than the suspect drug that could impact the signal. How strong is the drug – signal association?

Consistency of the data: Inconsistent data is a hindrance to arrive at a definite conclusion

Exposure response relationship: All angles of the exposure to the drug and occurrence of the event to be analyzed.

Biological plausibility: Is the condition reported medically reasonable or is it erroneous data.

Study findings: Take study findings into consideration

The nature and quality of the data: Are all relevant details reported or is it a scant report. What is the indication for the drug? Is it different in different countries? What is the indication being assessed.

Signal Management Process

Validation	– Data validation for factual accuracy.
Analysis	– Analysis of structured data to detect signals.
Prioritization	– Signal prioritization.
Evaluation	– In-depth assessment to finally confirm or refute signal.
Recommendation	– Action to be taken.
Implementation	– Implementation of the recommendation.

The focus during review of case reports initially can be on designated medical events (DME) and targeted medical events (TME).

Designated medical events are serious and rare events which have high drug-attributable possibility.

Targeted medical events are events of specific interest with regard to the drug.

Disproportionality-based Signal Detection Methods.

• Empirical Bayes multi-item gamma Poisson shrinker (MGPS)
• Proportional reporting ratio (PRR)

These perform differently with respect to the number and types of signals detected. In a comparative study it was reported that MPGS provides an objective and stable data.

A high-specificity disproportionality method combined with in depth medical analysis is the best way to conduct a quantitative and qualitative assessment.

The FDA has been trying out newer automated and rapid Bayesian data mining techniques to run through MedWatch. The data mining method, the Gamma Poisson Shrinker (GPS) program has now been replaced by the Multi-Item Gamma Poisson Shrinker (MGPS) program. The MGPS algorithm signal calculates not only for pairs, but also for combinations of drugs. Hence, events that are more frequent than just the drug – event pair associations are captured. MGPS minimizes random patterns and throws up consistent signals. The MGPS algorithm is also being evaluated to detect drug interactions and to detect differences among subgroups of gender and age. But MGPS cannot differentiate between known associations and new associations.

Signals of disproportionate reporting (SDR).

Statistical methods are particularly useful for analysis of large volume of ICSRs. Statistical methods identify and prioritize the signals. The next step is to analyze the additional factors and conduct an in-depth assessment to finally confirm or refute the signal.

Signals of disproportionate reporting (SDR) require evaluation of case reports, literature information, preclinical, pharmacological, pharmacoepidemiological and study data. Without statistical methods, analysis of such huge volume of data is just not possible.

Systematic Evaluation Of SDR

Signals of disproportionate reporting identified for further evaluation with statistical methods should be medically assessed. False positive results thrown up during statistical analysis have to be rejected. Statistical analysis currently has the disadvantage of not being able to thoroughly evaluate concomitant drug-event pairs and drug-drug interaction. These aspects as well as disease progression or concomitant disease has to be assessed by the medical reviewer. Combination of statistical methods with the classical method of in-depth review is the systematic evaluation of SDRs.

23. ARGUS

Oracle Argus Safety is the most widely used drug safety system in the world. This is a preferred option of small and large pharma companies to help them meet the reporting timelines and be compliant with regulatory guidelines.

Benefits of the Argus Safety Suite

• Both data management and regulatory reporting - Oracle Argus Safety provides an integrated querying and reporting application that supports management as well as regulatory reporting.

• A wide choice of data applications allows insightful data analysis.

• Integrated safety and risk management provides a comprehensive end-to-end solution.

• Single global database includes Japanese language.

Global annual safety reports for clinical and post-marketing surveillance are auto generated.

Case quality is through logical quality control checks as well as full source document integration.

Argus Safety takes a proactive approach to monitoring global regulatory updates and complies with all major regulatory reporting guideline such as the European Medicines Agency (EMEA), the U.S. Federal Drug Administration (FDA), and Japan's Pharmaceutical and Medical Devices Agency (PMDA).

Argus Safety incorporates the International Conference on Harmonization's current guidelines for transmitting data elements in individual case safety reports (ICH:E2B) which enables electronic exchange of information with partners and regulators without any hitch.

Drug Dictionary Access
MedDRA browser provides autoencoding capability

Argus Safety supports all standard dictionaries such as:
- Medical Dictionary for Regulatory Activities (MedDRA)
- Coding Symbols for a Thesaurus of Adverse Reaction Terms (CoSTART)
- World Health Organization Adverse Reactions Terminology (WHO-ART)
- World Health Organization Drug Dictionary (WHO-DRUG)
- International Classification of Diseases, Ninth Revision, Clinical Modification (ICD-9-CM)

Fully Integrated Safety System
Argus Safety seamlessly integrates with other products within the Argus product family. This provides the option of adding further functionality.

The following can be integrated with Oracle Argus Safety:
Oracle Argus Insight and Oracle Argus Perceptive - provide risk management analysis tools to ensure product analysis and decision making.

Oracle Argus Interchange - enables electronic exchange with partners and regulators. This allows integration with partners and to fully meet regulatory requirements in terms of timelines and guidelines.

Oracle Argus Affiliate - integrates affiliates and remote sites into the global workflow. This allows for seamless cohesion of the sponsor with its various branches across the globe. (LAM – Local Affiliate Module).

Oracle Argus Safety Japan - provides a full Japanese interface to each function in Oracle Argus Safety and includes specific compliance capabilities.

Oracle Argus Dossier - provides a collaboration platform to support the document writing process for periodic reports.

Oracle Argus Reconciliation - enables efficient reconciliation of data between clinical data systems and Oracle Argus Safety.

24. IMPORTANT MEDICAL EVENT

One of the first things you need to do when you receive a case is to determine whether the case is serious or non-serious. That can impact compliance and affect the sponsor financially as there is an implication for late regulatory submission.

Blood and Lymphatic System Disorders
Agranulocytosis
Aplasia
Aplastic anemia
Autoimmne - Hemolytic anemia, neutopenia, thrombocytopenia and pancytopenia
Blood dyscrasias including thrombocytopenia grade 3 and leucopenia grade 3
Bone marrow – Failure, toxicity, necrosis
Disseminated Intravascular Coagulation (DIC)
Hemolytic Anemia
Hemolytic Uremic Syndrome (HUS)
Pancytopenia
Thrombocytopenia - Idiopathic thrombocytopenia, thrombotic thrombocytic purpura and heparin induced thrombocytopenia (HIT)

Cardiac Disorders
Angina
Arrythmias
Asystole
Atrial Fibrillation
Atrial Flutter
Cardiac arrest
Cardiac tamponade
Cardiomyopathy
Cardiotoxicity
Carditis
Cardiac valve sclerosis
Cor Pulmonale
Coronary artery – aneurysm, dissection, perforation, insufficiency, embolism

Heart Failure
Ischemic Heart Disease
Left Ventricular failure
Myocarditis
Myocardial Infarction
Pericarditis
Pericardial effusion
Rhuematic heart disease
Right ventricular failure
Sick Sinus Syndrome
Torsades De Pointes
 Valve stenosis - Mitral, Pulmonary, Tricuspid
Ventricular tachycardia
Ventricular Fibrillation
Ventricular Flutter
Wolf Parkinson White syndrome

Congenital, Familial and Genetic Disorders
Congenital Anomalies
Porphyria

Ear and Labyrinth Disorders
Deafness – transitory, permanent, unilateral, conductive, neurosensory, mixed, sudden
Endolymphatic Hydrops
Haemotympanum
Meniere's disease
Ototoxicity

Endocrine Disorders
Acromegaly
Adrenal - Insufficiency, hemorrhage, suppression
Addison's disease
Addisonian crisis
Age related macular degeneration
Carcinoid syndrome
Cushing's syndrome
Diabetes

Diabetic Ketoacidosis
Gigantism
Glucocorticoid deficiency
Mineralocorticoid deficiency
Hyperammonaemic crisis
Toxic nodular goitre
Thyroiditis—Acute, autoimmune

Eye Disorders
Blindness – unilateral, transient, cortical
Cataract – cortical, diabetic
Chorioretinitis
Choroiditis
Conjunctival haemorrhage
Corneal – opacity, perforation
Eye haemorrhage
Glaucoma
Keratoconus
Optic Atrophy
Papilledema
Retinopathy
Retinal – detachment, degeneration, hemorrhage, dystrophy, oedema, ischaemia

Gastrointestinal Disorders
Acute Pancreatitis
Barett's oesophagus
Colitis
Duodenal Ulcer
Gastrointestinal haemorrhage
Haematemesis
Ileus
Intestinal Obstruction
Intussuception
Mallory Weiss Syndrome
Perforation
Peritonitis
Strangulated hernia
Volvulus

General Disorders and Administration Site Disorders
Hyperpyrexia (more than 40 deg C or 104 deg F)
Hypothermia
Multi-organ Failure
Multi-organ hypersensitivity Syndrome
Organ Failure
Pacemaker Syndrome
Stent embolisation

Hepatobiliary Disorders
Budd Chiari Syndrome
Cirrhosis
Hepatic Failure, Fibrosis, necrosis
Hepatitis
Hepatorenal Syndrome
Liver injury
Liver Sarcoidosis
Portal Hypertension
Reye Syndrome

Immune System Disorders
Anaphylactic Shock
Graft versus Host Disease
Neonatal myasthenia gravis
Polyarteritis Nodosa
Sarcoidosis
Transplant rejection

Infections and Infestations
Acquired immunodeficiency Syndrome (AIDS)
Bacteremia
Empyema
Endocarditis
Encephelitis
Gangrene
Haemorrhagic fever
Infective pericarditis
Meningitis
Myelitis

Osteomyelitis
Opportunistic Infections
Peritonitis
Sepsis
Septic Shock
Suspected transmission of an infectious agent by a drug
Tetanus
Tuberculosis

Injury
Accidental poisoning
Anesthetic complication — airway, cardiac, neonatal, pulmonary, vascular
Burns - 3rd and 4th degree
Brain herniation
Femur fracture
Hip Fracture
Heat Stroke
Spinal Cord injury
Uterine perforation

Investigations
ECG ST elevation and ST depression
Long QT syndrome
Prolonged QT

Musculoskeletal and connective tissue disorder
Bone Marrow Failure
Bone Infarction
Lymphoma
Malignant neoplasm
Myelodysplastic Syndrome
Osteonecrosis
Osteomalacia
Pathological fracture
Psoriatic arthropathy
Rhabdomyolysis
Rheumatoid arthritis
Systemic Lupus Erythematosis

Nervous System Disorders
Brain - Edema, injury, hypoxia, midline shift, compression
Cerebrovascular accident
Cerebral hemorrhage
Chiari (Arnold Chiari) malformation
Coma
Demyelinating disorders
Diabetic hyperosmolar coma
Encephelopathy
Extrapyramidal disorder
Hemiplegia
Hepatic encephalopathy
Hydrocephalus
Intracranial pressure increased
Myasthenia gravis
Multiple Sclerosis
Neuroleptic malignant syndrome
Optic neuritis
Prolonged loss of consciousnes
Seizures - New onset
Seizures aggravated
Status Epilepticus

Pregnancy and Perinatal Conditions
Abortion
Contraception failure (Oral, injectable and patch) resulting in pregnancy
Eclampsia
Ectopic pregnancy
Fetal Distress Syndrome
Fetal Growth retardation
Fetal death
Gestational Diabetes
HELLP Syndrome
Hemorrhage in pregnancy
Hydrops fetalis
Large for dates baby
Meconium in amniotic fluid

Oliogo and poly hydramnios
Placenta praevia
Placenta praevia hemorrhage
Pre-eclamsia
Premature baby
Premature separation of placenta
Small for dates baby
Still birth

Psychiatric Disorders
Acute psychosis
Anorexia nervosa
Bipolar disorder
Completed suicide
Delirium
Drug abuse
Drug dependence
Major depression
Suicidal behavior
Suicide attempt
Suicide ideation
Withdrawal Syndrome

Renal and Urinary Conditions
Acute renal failure
Anuria
Glomerulonephritis
Malignant renal hypertension
Nephrotic syndrome
Renal artery – occlusion, stenosis, thrombosis
Obstructive uropathy
Renal necrosis

Reproductive system and Breast Conditions
Azoospemia
Infertility
Ruptured Ovarian cyst
Uterine hemorrhage

Respiratory and thoracic condition
Acute respiratory distress syndrome
Acute respiratory failure
Anoxia
Alveolitis
Allergic alveolitis
Aspiration
Bronchospasm
Hemothorax
Hydrothorax
Hypoxia
Interstitial lung disease
Larngeal edema
Laryngospasm
Pneumothorax
Pulmonary embolism
Pulmonary fibrosis
Pulmonary hypertension
Respiratory failure, arrest, distress, depression
Status asthmaticus

Skin and Subcutaneous tissue condition
Alopecia totalis
Angioedema
Dermatitis bullous
Dermatitis exfoliative
Dermatitis exfoliative generalized
Drug reaction with eosinophilia and systemic symptoms (DRESS)
Erythema multiforme
Steven - Johnson syndrome
Toxic epidermal necrolysis

Vascular disorders
Aneurysm
Artery dissection
Circulatory collapse
Embolism
Hemorrhage

Hypertensive crisis
Infarction
Malignant hypertension
Shock - hemorrhagic, hypovolaemic
Thromboembolism
Thrombophlebitis
Thrombosis
Trousseau Syndrome
Vasculitis

25. NARRATIVE WRITING

Sample 1 A. Spontaneous Initial Report

A 36 year old patient called in to inform that he fell and broke his leg while he was weeding on 18 July 2013. He lived in Colarado,USA. He said "I am on the sponsor drug for 3 years for the treatment of generalised epilepsy." Earlier he was treated with phenobarbital which was stopped and he was then switched to the sponsor drug which he was currently taking. The dose of the film coated sponsor drug was 50mg daily. "And am also taking Norvasc for chronic hypertension." He has had migraine attacks since 5 years and 2 years ago he recalled having a seizure and being rushed to the ER where it was diagnosed as status epilepticus. He was treated with intravenous AED. Outcome: recovered. The patient said that this was not related to the sponsor drug. This report was received by the sponsor on 01-Jun-2013 by phone call. This is an initial report.

Narrative

This spontaneous report was received by the sponsor (name of the sponsor) from a consumer on 01-Jun-2013.

This concerns a currently 36 year old male patient from the United States of America. The medical history included migraine and chronic hypertension. The concomitant medication included Norvasc (amlodipine). The past drug included phenobarbital.

In 2010 the patient was initiated treatment with the sponsor drug (generic name)film coated tablet at a dose of 50 mg per day for the treatment of generalized epilepsy.

In 2011 the patient experienced an event of status epilepticus. Two years ago the patient had a seizure and he was rushed to the ER (emergency room) where he was diagnosed with status epilepticus. He was treated with intravenous AED (anti epileptic drug) and the event resolved.

On 18-Jul-2013 he fell and broke his leg.

The reporter assessed the causality of the event status epilepticus to the sponsor drug as not related.

At the time of the report, the event status epilepticus was resolved, the outcomes of the events fall and broke his leg were unknown and the sponsor drug was continued.

Rules Of Narrative Writing

• Identify the FRD (First Received Date) – The date when the initial report is received by the sponsor.

In this example: This is an initial report and was received by the sponsor on 01-Jan-2014. This is the first received date.

• Identify the suspect drug. The suspect drug can be one or more sponsor drugs and in addition one or more non-sponsor drugs.
In this example: The suspect drug is the sponsor drug. There is only one suspect drug in this case.

• Identify the past medical history from the event. The past medical history occurs prior to suspect drug initiation.
In this example: The suspect drug was started since 3 years. So, the events that occurred prior to 3 years are included in medical history.

• The event (adverse event) occurs after start of the suspect drug.
In this example: The adverse events that occur after start of the sponsor drug are the events.

• Write the narrative in chronological order - date wise.

• Any short forms should be written in full form
In this example: AED was reported in the source document. In the narrative this was written as AED (anti- epileptic drug)

• Brand names should be capitalized and generic for concomitant, past and suspect drugs should be in bracket.

Generics are always not capitalized.
Brand names are always capitalized.
In this example: Norvasc (amlodipine)

• At the end of the narrative, summarize the causality, action taken with suspect drug and outcome of the events.

Sample 1 B. Follow up Report

Follow up information was received on 30-Jun-2013. The consumer said that all events had resolved. He was also prescribed diclofenac for the broken leg pai.

Narrative

New relevant information was received from the consumer on 30-Jun-2013.
The patient had been prescribed diclofenac for the pain due to his broken leg.
At the time of report all events had resolved.

Rules Of Narrative Writing

• For follow up reports identify the LRD (Last Received Date) – The date the follow up report was received by the sponsor. This is the date from which the regulatory timelines are calculated.
In this example: The LRD is 30-Jun-2013.

Sample 2. Clinical Trial Report

Site number- 312 Subject number: 500098 Study : NA2105 DOB – 01-Jan-1971 Country: UK male.
Study Title: A multicenter, double blinded randomized controlled trial comparing the efficacy of sponsor drug comparator drug in long term treatment of type 2 diabetes mellitus in adults.

Event : STEMI Onset : 01-Jan-2014 Outcome: Resolving Causality: probable

Study drug : Comp/Sponsor drug – 200mg/10mg Route :oral From: 05-Feb-2009 Action taken : permanently discontinued on 02-Jan-2014. Treated with asprin for antiplatelet activity, nitroglycerin to relieve chest pain, and fibrinolytic therapy with streptokinase . No signs of cardiogenic shock.

Medical history: childhood infections, asthma. Concomitant medications: cetirizine for rhinitis & Duolin inhaler for asthma.

This report was received by fax on 05-Jan-2014

This interventional clinical trial report was received by the sponsor on on 05-Jan-2014.

This concerns a 43 year old male subject (312/500098) from United Kingdom. The medical history included childhood infections and asthma. The concomitant medications included cetirizine and Duolin (levosalbutamol and ipratropium bromide).

The subject was initiated treatment with the investigational drug from 05-Feb-2009, orally in the study NA2105 "A multicenter, double blinded randomized controlled trial comparing the efficacy of sponsor drug comparator drug in long term treatment of type 2 diabetes mellitus in adults" for the treatment of type 2 diabetes mellitus.

On 01-Jan-2014 he the subject had onset of ST elevation Myocardial Infarction (STEMI)

He was treated with aspirin for anti-platelet activity, nitroglycerin to relieve chest pain, and fibrinolytic therapy with streptokinase. He did not show signs of cardiogenic shock. The STEMI was resolving.

On 02-Jan-2014 the investigational drug was permanently discontinued.

The investigator assessed the causality of STEMI to the investigational drug as related.

At the time of report the event was resolving and the investigational drug was permanently discontinued.

Rules Of Narrative Writing.

• In report from study the patient is termed – subject

• In report from study the title of the study and the patient identifiers such as site/patient number should be included in the narrative.

• Treatment drugs are those which are started after the event and used for treating the patient. They should be mentioned along with the indication for which they are initiated.

• In this example: The treatment drugs and the indication are - Aspirin for anti-platelet activity, nitroglycerin to relieve chest pain, and fibrinolytic therapy with streptokinase.

• Concomitant medication is that which is used within 30 days of onset of event.
• Past drug is one that is used more than 30 days prior to onset of event.
We will use the above convention in this book. However be sure to find out the convention of the sponsor you are working for. It could be different.

GLOSSARY

Drug Abuse: Intentional excessive use of a drug on a occasional or consistent basis that results in harmful physical or psychological effects.

Drug Overdose: Administration of a dose or cumulative doses in a single day that is above the maximum recommended dose as per local labeling (SmPC or PI).

Drug Misuse: Drug is intentionally not used as per the prescription or as per recommendation with regards to dose, frequency, route or indication. Misuse also includes the use of prescription only drugs without prescription.

PI: Package Insert

Unsolicited reports: Those reports which are unsolicited by the sponsor. Spontaneous reports are unsolicited reports.

Off label: When the drug is not used as per the recommendations laid down in the local labeling – SmPC or the PI. Off label use could be for dose, route of administration, indication, population and others.

EPAR: European public assessment reports. The EMEA publishes an EPAR for every medicine granted a central marketing authorization by the European Commission following an assessment by the EMA's Committee for Medicinal Products for Human Use (CHMP). EPARs are full scientific assessment reports of medicines authorized at a European Union level.

DSUR: Development Safety Update report. The DSUR is an annual report which includes safety data from all clinical trials conducted with the investigational drug using all indications, all dosage forms, and all intended populations. The data lock point (DLP) for a DSUR is based on the date of the first authorization to conduct interventional clinical trials in any country (DIBD). The DSUR is submitted annually to regulatory authorities within 60 days from the DIBD.

PADER: Periodic adverse drug experience report and the PAER - Periodic adverse experience report for the USA. These are in the advanced stage of being replaced by the PBRER for the US FDA.

AR: Aggregate Reporting. Aggregate reporting involves the compilation of safety data and reporting these as per the required formats within a specified time limit set using the DLP. The aggregate reporting for a drug occurs over a prolonged period of time running into years.

DIBD: Development International Birth Date - the date of the first authorization to conduct interventional clinical trials in any country.

CIOMS: Council for International Organizations of Medical Sciences.

IIS: investigator Initiated Study

Pre - treatment case: Subject signs the informed consent form and joins the study but had adverse events even prior to being randomized. Such cases in which events occur even before the investigational drug is started are termed as pre-treatment cases.

Lack of Efficacy (LOE): Failure of a drug to produce the intended therapeutic benefit or pharmacological action.

INN: International Non proprietary Name

Courtesy Cases: Cases which are received by a sponsor from other pharma company conducted studies in which the sponsor's drug is involved.

AESI: Adverse events of special interest. Toxicology profile and other nonclinical data may lead to possible toxicities that could potentially occur in humans. Based on this, knowledge of the underlying disease and the mechanism of action of the investigational drug, it is decided that certain adverse events that occur after starting the investigational drug are termed as Adverse Events of Special Interest (AESI). AESI is a potential risk and requires increased surveillance. AESI require special collection or reporting - detailed follow-up and prompt reporting to the sponsor.

AESM: Adverse event of special monitoring.

AEFI: Adverse event following immunization.

QOW: Every other week.

QW: Every week.

THE PHARMACOVIGILANCE INTERVIEW

THE PHARMACOVIGILANCE INTERVIEW

Q.1) The following are software based pharmacovigilance safety applications
A. Oracle Argus.
B. Oracle AERS.
C. Aris G
D. Empirica Trace
E. All the above

Q.2) Match the following regulatory authorities with their country.
Swiss Medic
Bfarm,
MHLW
CDSCO
MHRA
LAREB
Afsaapps / ANSM
TGA
SFDA
China, Switzerland, India, U.K, Japan, Sweden, France, Germany, Australia,Netherland.

Q.3) Pfizer, Novartis, Merck, Bristol Mayers Squibb, GSK Pharma, Amgen, Roche, Novo Nordisk are names of Sponsors
A. True
B. False

Q.4) Fill in the blanks.
Regulatory Timelines :
A. Within ------- days for SAE (serious adverse event)
B. Within ------- days Clinical Trial DLT (Death & Life threatening)
C. Within _____ days for spontaneous DLT (Death & Life threatening)

Q.5)　What is Black Box warning?

Q.6)　_____ is the

Q.8)　Vol 9A is replaced by _____

Q 9)　Submission in ICH E2B (R2) format to EudraVigilance will be changed to----------------------

Q 10)　CCSI stands for --

Q11)　A pharmacist reported that Mrs C had gum hypertrophy. Can this be a valid case?

Q.12)　The following statements are TRUE or FALSE?

a.　A patient or his relative can report adverse events to the drug regulatory authority or the company. This is called spontaneous report.

b.　A patient or his relative can report adverse events to the Drug Regulatory Authority's Pharmacoviglance Programme by phone, fax, email or website.

c.　National regulatory authorities who are members of the WHO International Drug Monitoring Programme, submit reports to the Uppsala Monitoring Centre in Sweden - the world bank of adverse events.

d.　Cases need to be reported even if all details regarding the events are unavailable

e.　Cases need to be reported if it is not sure that the events are caused by the drug itself.

f.　The CIOMS-I form is the standard form for expedited reporting of adverse events.

g.   Spontaneous reports have implied causality.

h.   Implied causality is based on the belief that if the reporter has taken time to send across a report then it means he is doing so because he believes there is some sort of causality between the suspect and the events.

I.   Reporting an adverse event does not necessarily mean that there is a definite link between the event and the product.

j.   Spontaneous report is an unsolicited report.

k.   Clinical trial report is a solicited report.

l.   Drug exposure in utero occurs in a baby.

m.   Drug exposure during pregnancy occurs in a mother.

n.   The Last Received Date is the Day Zero. The day the sponsor first receives the initial report.

o.   The Last Received Date is the Day Zero. The day the sponsor first receives the follow up report.

p.   Spontaneous reporting is important for conducting the risk-benefit analysis of new drugs.

Q 13)
a.   Off label use for dose: When prescribed by the doctor or used by the patient the dose is more than the company recommended dose.

b.   Off label use for population: When the drug for instance is used in a child when the company recommends its use only in adults.

c.   Pregnancy reports are of 2 types – retrospective and prospective.

d.   A pregnancy report is Prospective when the pregnancy is ongoing

e. A pregnancy report is Retrospective when the outcome of the pregnancy – delivery of the baby, miscarriage/abortion has happened at the time of report.

f. A pregnancy report is Retrospective when pregnancy is ongoing but it is known for instance, through sonography that the fetus has a congenital anomaly.

g. An event can have these possible outcomes: Fatal, life- threatening, resolved with sequelae, not resolved, resolved and unknown.

h. The term "severe" refers to the intensity of an event. A severe event need not be a seriousevent.

I. In cases where a withdrawal reaction is experienced, a dechallenge is when the drug is again given to the patient.

j. Rechallenge happens only on positive dechallenge.

k. On rechallenge in some cases the reaction may be more severe.

l. Rechallenge is done rarely, since the benefit of reintroducing the drug to the patient has to be weighed against the risk of recurrence of the reaction.

m. For not yet approved medicinal product a company's Investigator's Brochure will serve as the source document to assess the expectedness of an event.

n. Ideally, even if unblinding is required, the blind should be maintained for biometrics personnel and for those responsible for analysis and interpretation of study results.

o. Serious, related and unexpected reactions associated with placebo (a reaction due to an excipient), result in a SUSAR and should be reported by the sponsor.

p. Before reporting SUSAR unblinding should be carried out.

Q.14)

a. Biological products include a wide range of products such as vaccines, blood and blood component s, Issues , and recombinant therapeutic proteins.

b. The Center for Biologics Evaluation and Research (CBER) is responsible for ensuring the safety and efficacy of biological products.

c. Biologics are used in the treatment of autoimmune and inflammatory diseases such as rheumatoid arthritis, psoriatic arthritis, ankylosing spondylitis, Crohn's disease.

d. Merck is associated with J/J-Johnson & Johnson blockbuster biologic Remicaide (infliximab).

e. Biologics have an increased risk of life-threatening infection, occurrence of cancer and cardiovascular risk among elderly patients.

f. Rituxan from Roche is a non-anti-TNF best selling cancer drug. It is also used in treatment of first line anti-TNF drugs such as Humira, Enbrel or Remicaide.

g. New legislation may allow for generic companies to manufacture biosimilars.

Q.15)

a. FDA's Center for Drug Evaluation and Research (CDER) Office of Generic Drugs, is the regulatory authority for Abbreviated New Drug Application (ANDA).

b. An ANDA application for generics does not require both preclinical and clinical trials to be done. This saves several years and huge amount of funds for the generic company.

c. ANDA applicants should demonstrate that their product is bioequivalent by performing BA and BE studies.

d. Bioequivalence: When Bioavailability of generic is ____ to ____ % of Bioavailability of the innovator.

e. A generic drug is similar to an innovator drug in dosage form, strength, route of administration, and indication.

f. The Orange Book contains all approved and generic drugs in USA.

g. Information regarding a possible causal relationship between an adverse event and a drug, the relationship being previously unknown or incomplete is a signal.

h. Generally more than a single report is required to generate a signal.

I. Signal Detection is part of advanced pharmacovigilance.

j. Signal Detection is the first alert and indicates that further evaluation is required.

k. PASS - Post authorization safety study is conducted to assess the safety risk of an authorized medicinal product

l. WHO International Drug Monitoring Centre (IDMC) is located at Uppsala, Sweden.

m. It is mandatory for the sponsor to report cases only from the sponsor funded websites.

n. Haemovigilance is vigilance of transfusion-related adverse events.

o. Materiovigilance is vigilance of medical devices related adverse events

p. Monitoring Drug Safety is also useful for licensee or generic manufacturer as they can assess the safety advantages of drugs.

q. Hosting of databases by means of cloud computing is gaining increased acceptance in the industry.

r. With regard to the content and format of electronic ICSRs, marketing authorization holders should adhere to the internationally agreed : ICH M1 terminology - Medical Dictionary for Regulatory Activities (MedDRA).

Q. 16) PSUR is replaced by --------- by the EMEA.

Q. 17) The CFR—code of federal regulations has 50 titles. Section 21 of the CFR is regarding food and drugs regulations.

Q 18) Fill in the blanks.
       21 CFR 11 _____
       21 CFR 50 _____
       21 CFR 56 _____
       21 CFR 201 _____
       21 CFR 312 _____
       21 CFR 314 _____
       21 CFR 316 _____

Q.19) Deciding whether a case is serious or non serious can impact regulatory compliance

Q. 20) In MedDRA, for the major SOC such as cardiac, hepatic, pulmonary, and renal the words "failure" and "insufficiency" treated as synonyms. The term "insufficiency" at the LLT is coded to the PT term "failure": LLT - Renal insufficiency PT - Renal Failure. Is this True?

Q. 21)

a) Can there be more than one suspect drug?

b) An HIV patient on anti - HIV drugs dies. Will you code for Lack of Efficacy?

c) Can a suspect drug be a non-sponsor (other company drug)?

d) If lack of efficacy is associated with a serious adverse event it is an expedited reportable case for EMEA.

e) If lack of efficacy is associated with a serious and unexpected adverse event it is an expedited reportable case for FDA.

f) The FDA recognizes that privacy is an important concern. The information and reporter's identity will not be given out in public.

g) MedDRA is updated twice every year in the months of March and September.

h) When a medicinal product is new to the market and only a small number of ICSRs have been received, it is more feasible to assess these ICSRs individually than to use statistical methods. The reliability of the statistical screening is limited by the small numbers of ICSRs.

I) The current statistical methods only operate with a limited number of data fields that are related mainly to the drug-event pair and the patient's characteristics. Experience with regard to the extensive ICH E2B(M) and M2 data fields is required in order to further advance the scope and output of statistical methods.

J) Pharmacovigilance data-mining algorithms (DMAs) such as the urn-model based algorithm, the Gamma Poisson Shrinker (GPS) and proportional reporting ratio (PRR), are known to generate significant numbers of false-positive signals of disproportionate reporting (SDRs),

22) Report Through MedWatch:

The MedWatch form can be used to report adverse events of drugs for human use, drug side effects, drug use errors, product quality complaint, and therapeutic failures for:

• Prescription or over-the-counter medicines, at the hospital or at the outpatient clinic.

- Biologics (such as blood components, blood and plasma derivatives, allergenic, human cells, tissues used for transplantation (tendons, ligaments, and bone)

- Medical devices (including in vitro diagnostic products)

- Combination drugs

- Special nutritional supplements or foods (dietary supplements, infant formulas, and medical foods)

- Cosmetics

- Foods and beverages

23) Steps Of Signal Detection

Signal Identification

Literature search

Initial Data Analysis

Additional information from various sources

Consult with the WHO Centre for International Drug Monitoring and Sponsor

Final Data Analysis and Conclusion

Detailed report

24)
a. Periodic safety reports: This allows for an ongoing assessment of whether the therapeutic benefit of the drug justifies the risk.

b. Only serious and unexpected cases have to be reported on an expedited basis to US FDA.

c.   GVP Module XV -- appropriate communication of relevant safety information to healthcare professionals and patients.

d.   GVP Module XII - product information is kept up-to-date with the current scientific knowledge and relevant authorities are kept upto date including communication on new or changed risks.

e.   GVP Module VI - Management and reporting of adverse drug reactions

f.   GVP Module IX - Signal management

25)
a.   FDA defines   "Soft Coding" as – Selecting a term which is both less specific and less severe.

b.   One condition is more specific than the other. This is an important consideration in MedDRA Coding.

c.   Prescription errors – When doctors do not follow the sponsor's recommendations as laid down in the SmPC or PI.

d.   Syndactyly is a serious case requiring expedited reporting.

e.   Regulatory timeline for interventional clinical trial is 7 days.

Q.1) E.

Q.2)

Swissmedic	==	Switzerland
BfArM	==	Germany
MHLW	==	Japan. Ministry of Health, Labour and Welfare
CDSCO	==	India. Central Drug Standards Control Organization
MHRA	==	U. K. Medicines and health care products regulatory agency
LAREB	==	Sweden. Landelijke Registratie Evaluatie Bijwerkingen
Afsaapps	==	France.
SFDA	==	China. State Food and Drug Administration
HSA	==	Singapore. Health Sciences Authority
TGA	==	Australia. Therapeutic Goods Administration

Q.3) A.

Q.4)
A.15 days
B.7 days
C.15 days

Q. 5) FDA Boxed Warning
The "black box warning." is used on the labeling information of prescription drugs if they have potential serious or life-threatening risk profile.

Q.6)   EUDRALEX

Q.7)   Vol 9 A

Q.8)   GVP

Q.9)   E2B (R3)

Q.10)   Company Core Safety Information.

Q.11).   There are 4 components for MSI. Here, the drug is missing and hence this is not a valid case.

Q 12)   a-p. All statements are True.

Q 13)   a-p. All statements are True.

Q 14)   a-g. All statements are True.

Q 15)   a-r. All statements are True.

d.   Bioequivalence: When Bioavailability of generic is 80 to 125 % of Bioavailability of the innovator.

Q 16)   PBRER

Q 17)   True

Q.18).
    21 CFR 11 - Electronic records and signatures
    21 CFR 50 - Protection of human subjects
    21 CFR 56 - Institutional Review Board
    21 CFR 201 - Drug labeling
    21 CFR 312 - Investigational New Drug Application
    21 CFR 314 - New Drug Application
    21 CFR 316 - Orphan drugs

Q.19)   True

Q.20)   True.

Q.21)
a.   Yes
b.   No. LOE has not been reported.
c-j . True

Q.22 -Q. 25. True

SERIOUS OR NON-SERIOUS

1. A patient with Thyroid Nodule

2. A patient is on anticoagulants. Laboratory tests reveal an INR of 3

3. A physician reports ear perforation associated with pain in one of his patients.

4. A consumer report by the patient's sibling informs of weight loss of 12.5 kilograms in a month. The baseline weight was 100 kilograms

5. A registered nurse reports from a clinic about a patient who had brain injury

6. A lady has had breast lump removal

7. A consumer report mentions of an accident in which two patients suffered injury. One patient had concussion

8. A consumer report mentions of an accident in which two patients suffered injury. One patient had concussion associated with loss of consciousness for quite some time.

9. A pharmacist reports a case of serum sickness 10. A consumer reports allergic bronchospasm

11. An intravenous medication was given intramuscularly by mistake and the patient was taken to the emergency room. She was treated and discharged after a few hours.

12. A nurse reports neutropenia in a patient

13. Withdrawal Syndrome

14. Withdrawal Symptoms of itching and headache

15. A HCP reports excessive birth weight of the baby

16. A HCP reports low birth weight of the baby (less than 2.5kg)

17. Unintended pregnancy and condom failure pregnancy

18. Talipes

19. Spina bifida

20. An unintended pregnancy after hormonal contraceptive failure and while on intrauterine device (IUD)

21. LOE of an oral contraceptive, LOE of a drug used for treatment of life threatening disease and LOE of a vaccine

22. Congenital anomaly

23. Borderline Steven – Johnson Syndrome

ANSWER

1. Non-serious. Most thyroid nodules are benign. And there is nothing in the report to suggest it is cancerous.

2. Non –serious. 2.5 x 1.5 (Two and half times the baseline) is the calculation. Since an INR of 3 is less than this it is considered non serious. The INR is typically used to monitor patients on warfarin or related oral anticoagulant therapy. A high INR indicates risk of bleeding.

3. Ear perforation (ruptured tympanic membrane) associated with pain is a non-serious case. It tends to become serious if associated with loss of hearing (temporary or permanent disability).

4. Serious

5. Serious

6. Breast lump is considered benign (unless otherwise reported). Hence this is a non-serious report.

7. Concussion is a MBTI (mild brain traumatic injury) and is a non serious case.

8. Serious. Concussion associated with repeated vomiting, loss of consciousness for quite some time or deterioration of consciousness is a serious case.

9. Non-serious

10. Serious

11. Medication error – non-serious.

12. Unless specified as neutropenia grade 3 or 4 it is a non-serious case.

13. Serious

14. Non serious

15. Serious

16. Serious

17. Non serious

18. Serious

19. Serious.

20. Serious.

21. Serious.

22. Serious.

23. Serious.

24. Serious.

25. Serious.

THUMB RULES

Non-Serious

INR - 4. On anticoagulants an INR upto 4

Weight gain/loss upto 10% per month of baseline

Weight gain/loss upto 25% a year of the baseline

Grade 1 and 2 Neutropenia

Grade 1 and 2 thrombocytopenia

THINKABOUT IT

Opportunistic infection in a drug with immunosuppression listed in the RSI. Is this a serious or non-serious case?

Fungal infection, herpes zoster infection in a drug with immunosuppression listed in the RSI.

Drug is contraindicated for renal failure.

Should this be off label for population or indication?

About Physician.

Qualified in clinical research.
Experienced in pharmacovigilace.
Medical Approver & Quality Lead for ICSR's submitted to
USA - FDA, EMEA and Japan- MHLW.
Pharmacovigilance trainer.

Corporate career
Apollo, Manipal, Mphasis & Accenture

Dr. RaviN Humbarwadi

SPONSOR

DR. NSH FOUNDATION
Surgeon Par Excellence
www.drnsh.com

PRANAV PUBLICATIONS
Audio, television, animation enquiries
contact ralah09@gmail.com
Mobile: 9686933749

Notes

Notes

Notes

Notes

Notes

Notes

Notes

Notes

Notes

Notes

Notes

Notes

E CTD

The electronic common technical document (e CTD) provides guidance related to the electronic submission of applications for human pharmaceutical products. The eCTD has guidelines for regulatory submissions of new drug applications (ANDAs), biologics license applications (BLAs), investigational new drug applications (INDs), new drug application (NDAs), master files such as drug master files, advertising material and promotional labeling.

This guidance to the industry clarifies where the integrated summary of effectiveness (ISE) and integrated summary of safety (ISS) are to be included in the common technical document (CTD) format. The ISE and ISS are not just summaries but actually detailed integrated analyses of all relevant data from the clinical study reports.

E CTD considers the ISE and ISS to be critical components of the clinical efficacy and safety portions of a marketing or licensing application. Therefore, the ISE and ISS should be generally placed in Module 5, section 5.3.5.3. If the narrative portion of the ISE or ISS is suitable for use in section 2.7.3 or 2.7.4, the narrative portion should be submitted only once and referenced in both Module 2 (section 2.7.3 or 2.7.4) and Module 5, section 5.3.5.3

The documents, whether for a marketing application or an investigational application should be organized based on the five modules in the CTD:

Module 1 includes administrative information and prescribing information

Module 2 includes CTD summary documents

Module 3 includes information on quality

Module 4 includes the nonclinical study reports

Module 5 includes the clinical study reports

Electronic Common Technical Document.

Electronic submission to the FDA first started in 01-Jan-2008.

Electronic submissions will be mandatory in the future. Specialized software is required to format documents for eCTD submission. It has been proposed that twenty four months after publishing the final guidance document all new NDA and all new BLA submissions need to be through eCTD.

Become A Film Producer

Salt n Pepper has excellent stories and scripts for animation.

Random Boys

The Sci- fi Project

The General and the Teknologist

Contact: ralah09@gmail.com

Donate For A Cause

Dr. NSH FOUNDATION
A charitable hospital for the needy

Contact: ralah09@gmail.com

www.ingramcontent.com/pod-product-compliance
Lightning Source LLC
Chambersburg PA
CBHW051809170526
45167CB00005B/1945